CARDIOVASCULAR HEALTH

CARDIOVASCULAR HEALTH

How Conventional Wisdom Is Failing Us

Jay N. Cohn

ROWMAN & LITTLEFIELD
Lanham • Boulder • New York • London

Published by Rowman & Littlefield
A wholly owned subsidary of The Rowman & Littlefield Publishing Group, Inc.
4501 Forbes Boulevard, Suite 200, Lanham, Maryland 20706
www.rowman.com

Unit A, Whitacre Mews, 26-34 Stannary Street, London SE11 4AB

British Library Cataloguing in Publication Information Available

Library of Congress Cataloging-in-Publication Data

Names: Cohn, Jay N., author.
Title: Cardiovascular health : how conventional wisdom is failing us / Jay N. Cohn.
Description: Lanham : Rowman & Littlefield, [2017] | Includes bibliographical references and index.
Identifiers: LCCN 2017001845 (print) | LCCN 2017003021 (ebook) | ISBN 9781442275126 (cloth :
    alk. paper) | ISBN 9781442275133 (Electronic)
Subjects: | MESH: Cardiovascular Diseases--genetics | Cardiovascular Diseases--prevention &
    control
Classification: LCC RC682 (print) | LCC RC682 (ebook) | NLM WG 120 | DDC 616.1/2042--dc23
LC record available at https://lccn.loc.gov/2017001845

∞ ™ The paper used in this publication meets the minimum requirements of
American National Standard for Information Sciences—Permanence of Paper for
Printed Library Materials, ANSI/NISO Z39.48-1992.

Printed in the United States of America

CONTENTS

INTRODUCTION

Advice about health care saturates the media these days. Newspapers, magazines, radio, and TV as well as the Internet are responding to the fascination of the public with understanding threats to their health and ways to deal with them. The commercials during prime-time TV are dominated by ads for obscure new drugs that advise people to "ask your doctor" about prescribing them. Despite the apparent narrow target for these expensive commercials, they wouldn't exist unless they were effective in generating considerable revenue for the sponsors. I have suspected that they only appear if the drug company is having trouble penetrating the medical market.

People are also warned about their personal risk of developing severe, life-threatening illnesses and what they can do to reduce their chance of getting sick or dying. Whether it is what to eat, what to do, or what to think, the advice is often based on studies in large populations using large databases that are increasingly available for analysis. Such large databases are generated by hospitals; health-care-provider groups; insurance companies; local, state, and federal government agencies; and even some countries. Although the accuracy of these databases is not always assured, they provide individual investigators with a powerful tool to evaluate relationships in that specific population between various measurements or entries in the records.

For instance, the data may demonstrate an association between some trait, such as obesity, defined by a body mass index over 30 kg/m2, and the likelihood of developing a disease such as a heart attack. The obligatory statistical exercise in such studies is to search for some other difference in those individuals with and without the trait of interest that could account for a different rate of the disease. Is the population with or without the trait older, more sedentary, poorer, less educated, and so on? If no other differences are found, the investigators might conclude that the difference is related to the trait of interest. What is often left unsaid is that the investigators can only examine differences on which they have collected data. A host of potential hereditary and environmental factors always remain unexamined. So the association is at best worthy of a hypothesis, not a conclusion.

If the observation is replicated in another population, the association between the trait and the outcome may be real and statistically sound, but the meaning of this association for an individual is often hardly discernible. The difference between population data on health and individual health is usually blurred by the media as well as by the scientists who promulgate such data. Population data—that acquired by studying a large group of individuals, regardless of how they are selected—applies only modestly and variably to any given individual. Some of these observations are reproducible and real and should be taken seriously, but many are of little importance and probably should be disregarded.

Even if an association is demonstrated, and even if it is verified by repeating the observation in another population, the lay medical reports often err by inappropriately assuming cause and effect. These reporters, and sometimes even the scientists, are willing to suggest that the reported behavior or trait is responsible for the reported outcome, such as an excess of sickness or death. But cause and effect can never be gleaned from an association. I am reminded of an experience from more than forty years ago. A prominent medical journal published a rather unusual observation that people with earlobe creases have a higher risk of heart attacks than those without earlobe creases.[1] These creases were shown on a photograph of a man who had a diagonal crease or line running across the lower portion of his ear lobe. I received calls from several patients who, alarmingly having noted that they had such creases, asked if they could come in to have the creases removed. How naïve, I thought at the time, that people might think that removing the creases would reduce their risk of a heart attack. Certainly people should have known that an association, which might imply some similar condition affecting the earlobe or an inherited trait somehow linked to both the creases and coronary artery disease, is different than true cause and effect. There certainly is no basis for even entertaining the idea that an earlobe crease could cause heart attacks or that their removal would decrease the risk. To prove cause and effect, one would need to carry out a prospective trial of randomly assigning such individuals to surgical removal or no surgical removal to determine if removing the creases reduced the risk. The medical profession has unfortunately carried out many futile trials in recent years, but no scientist would embark on such a silly endeavor. It makes no sense. There must be a rational mechanism for the effect to justify a trial. Association is not equivalent to cause and effect.

Certainly physicians would be able to properly advise their patients, you might think. But doctors don't always think clearly about cause and effect. They too are bombarded with the news media and their professional organizations that preach the party line. Often this party line blurs the distinction between association and cause and effect. Yes, obese individuals have a higher risk of heart attacks than thin ones, but are we certain that when the obese person loses weight, the risk returns to normal? Not really, though it is a reasonable and testable hypothesis. Such a study hasn't been done because of its difficulty. It would require studying thousands of patients and trying to convince half of them to lose weight, but not the other half that would serve as the control group. They would need to be followed for a number of years to determine if the rate of heart attacks in the weight-loss group—if indeed they actually lost weight—was lower than that in the control group. It would be a monstrously expensive study to perform and highly unlikely to be successful. Who would be interested in funding it?

Lay and scientific articles also often fail to distinguish between relative risk and absolute risk. For example, the American Heart Association has reviewed large population data noting that there may be a lower risk of heart attacks in pet owners compared to non–pet owners.[2] The data are certainly not very persuasive, and the magnitude of effect, if there really is an effect, is very difficult to calculate. But let's accept that there is an effect, and let's even assume that the effect is remarkably large, like a 20 percent reduction in heart attacks or even deaths from heart disease. That is a relative risk reduction. Twenty percent fewer individuals with a pet got a heart attack than those without a pet. That certainly doesn't mean that going out and buying a pet will reduce your risk because that association could have multiple mechanisms, including the personality trait that chooses to have a pet, the walking that pet owners are obligated to undertake, the comfort of having an adoring "friend," or some other lifestyle factor shared by pet owners. Even if pet ownership did reduce the relative risk by a whopping 20 percent, a number that makes us take notice, the absolute risk reduction is really quite modest. Suppose you had two chances in 100 of having a heart attack in the next ten years and pet ownership (please note that we do not even know if pet ownership is responsible) reduced that risk by 20 percent. That would reduce your risk from 2 percent in ten years to 1.6 percent in ten years, a pretty unimpressive benefit. The absolute risk reduction is only 0.4 percent over ten years. This makes the apparent benefit or harm of any activity for any individual pretty unimpressive. Even if the observation could be documented in other large population bases, it could not justify anyone acquiring a dog for protection against heart attacks.

Another conceptual weakness of the medical profession is its dependence on diagnostic categories. Everything has to have a name. An office visit or a hospitalization requires a diagnosis. Reimbursement to doctors and hospitals is dependent on the name of the condition being treated. Even diagnostic uncertainty may be rewarded with a label. For example, "fever of unknown origin" is an official diagnostic code.

This dedication to a diagnostic label leads to a comfort level in the medical caregiver and in the patient. It satisfies insurance companies. It provides the opportunity for textbooks, journal articles, and treatment guidelines to discuss diagnostic tests, treatment, and prognosis. It allows health-care organizations to analyze all their experience with a specific diagnostic condition. It is how caregivers communicate with each other.

But this quest for diagnostic homogeneity can be misleading. Many diagnostic categories present as rather arbitrary thresholds of continuous variables. The American Psychiatric Association has recently changed the diagnostic criteria for autism and its associated disorders.[3] There are no rigid diagnostic criteria for autism, merely behavioral differences that are on a continuum from what society views as normal to grossly abnormal. Where is the threshold for the diagnosis set? If too low, many might be inappropriately captured into a disease category. If too high, behavioral services may become unavailable for many who could benefit. Parents and schools are having similar problems with the diagnostic criteria and treatment of so-called attention deficit hyperactivity disorder. Where does normal end and abnormal begin?

Everyone has a blood pressure, but only when it is higher than a threshold of 140/90 mmHg does one get labeled as having "hypertension." If your blood pressure is 136/86 mmHg, should you be reassured? That 4 mmHg difference is barely discernible by the blood pressure device, and the reading varies each time it is taken. But guidelines tell the doctor to treat 140/90 but not 136/86 mmHg. Is that rational?

Fasting blood sugar levels vary widely among patients, but only when they are higher than an arbitrary threshold of 126 mg% does the individual get labeled as having "diabetes." Is a blood sugar of 120 mg% really much different? Even the more contemporary measurement of hemoglobin A1C, which serves as a more stable guide to blood sugar levels over time, has an arbitrary threshold for normalcy. Similarly, blood cholesterol and lipid levels are used to define a diagnostic category called "hyperlipidemia," but the absolute level of these fats in the blood that justifies this diagnosis is controversial. Obesity has been labeled as a disease by the American Heart Association. Its definition is, of course, arbitrary, whether based on weight or body mass index or even waist circumference. There is no rigorous line with any of these variables between normal and abnormal. I will discuss each of these "diseases" in the chapters that follow.

Even the diagnosis of cancer has in recent years been the subject of controversy. Does a single so-called malignant cell or a small group of cells identified as malignant on a biopsy justify the diagnosis of cancer? We now know that many of these lesions in the breast and prostate never lead to invasive cancer and thus probably shouldn't be so labeled. Diagnoses are therefore often misleading and may result in inappropriate therapy that can be more harmful than the so-called diseases they are designed to treat.

For health-care providers, placing patients into diagnostic categories provides them with the comfort of following guidelines for management. It serves as a safe harbor in the rough sea of uncertainty. It allows them to stop thinking and start treating. Once the patient can be fit into the box of the disease process, the rest is rather straightforward. Caregivers know the proper treatment and the therapeutic target. Or, as we shall explore in the pages that follow, do they?

A corollary to comfort with a diagnosis is comfort with traditional ideas, especially if these conventional ideas have long driven a doctor's approach to health care. The medical and lay press has hammered for years on risk factors as a cause of cardiovascular diseases such as heart attacks and strokes. Risk factors include those measurements that fulfill the criteria for the diagnosis of hypertension, hyperlipidemia, obesity, and diabetes. Thus the conventional view is that preventing heart attacks is a process of preventing risk factors from developing and treating them if they appear. Health-care providers who rigorously apply the guidelines can be comfortable that they are doing everything asked of them.

Then why have we had such modest success in preventing heart attacks and strokes? Guidelines for treatment of these risk factors are based on clear evidence for the effectiveness of therapy in preventing these morbid events. The physiological and pathological mechanisms of these morbid events are pretty thoroughly understood. These events are clearly preventable. Then why haven't we succeeded in eliminating them? Are the risk factors being inadequately treated? Perhaps. But more importantly, as we will discuss, the diagnostic categories leave many individuals who are at high risk out of the treatment guidelines. Failure to achieve the diagnostic criteria for a treatable level of a risk factor does not at all mean the absence of risk. Treatment is being withheld from many because they don't fit into our comfortable diagnostic categories. And medical practitioners, steeped in conventional thinking, fail to identify the bulk of individuals who are tomorrow's heart attack victims.

The goal of this book is to explore the current state of medical knowledge regarding blood pressure, cholesterol, blood sugar, obesity, diet, exercise, and other risk factors for the occurrence of cardiovascular morbid events. We will find that conventional thinking, which continues to dominate medical education, may be contributing to the persistently high rates of heart attacks and other cardiovascular illnesses. I also will propose a solution to the problem.

I

WHAT CAUSES HEART ATTACKS, STROKES, AND OTHER CARDIOVASCULAR ILLNESSES?

CONVENTIONAL WISDOM

- Heart attacks occur because of a sudden and unpredictable blockage of a coronary artery that nourishes the heart muscle.
- Strokes occur because of a sudden and unpredictable blockage or rupture of an artery nourishing the brain.
- Heart attacks and strokes are largely the consequence of an unhealthy lifestyle.
- Sudden death is a consequence of an unpredictable electrical abnormality of the heart rhythm, sometimes the first sign of coronary artery disease that leads to heart attacks.
- Blockage of the circulation to the legs is an inevitable complication of aging.
- Kidney failure and dementia are diseases of aging that are not due to artery or heart disease.
- Diabetes results from being overweight and eating too much carbohydrate.

WHAT IS CARDIOVASCULAR DISEASE?

The heart and the blood vessels constitute the cardiovascular system. They contain the circulating blood that nourishes all the tissues and organs of the body. The left ventricle of the heart pumps the blood into the arteries, which deliver the blood to all the tissues. The veins collect the blood from the tissues and return it to the heart, where it is replenished with oxygen from the lungs and repumped at about one-second intervals. This finely honed system is vital to our health, allowing all our organs to function and providing oxygen to our muscles during exercise and to our brain when we think.

The concept of cardiovascular disease is difficult to define. Is it present only when the arteries fail to deliver the blood supply needed or when the heart is not able to pump adequately to support the organs of the body? There is no question that these symptomatic conditions warrant the designation "cardiovascular disease." If the heart muscle is critically deprived of blood flow, chest pain develops. If the brain is deprived of adequate blood flow, there may be paralysis of limbs, speech impairment, or loss of consciousness. If the kidney loses its blood supply, waste products accumulate in the body instead of being excreted in the urine. If the legs are deprived of blood supply, pain develops and the legs become pale and cool. If the heart pumping ability is impaired, there is fatigue and shortness of breath. These are certainly signs of cardiovascular disease.

But what about earlier stages of the disease, before symptoms appear? What about when the arteries are beginning to get clogged but they have not yet critically obstructed blood flow? What if the heart's pumping ability is getting impaired but the patient is not yet aware of any symptoms? If these abnormalities could be detected, should we label them as cardiovascular disease? If we knew these abnormalities were destined to progress to symptomatic disease, then it would be appropriate to label them as an early stage of cardiovascular disease. If treatment could prevent that progression—and prevention at that early stage would be far more effective than treatment instituted after symptoms develop—then it would be particularly important to search for, identify, and treat these early stages of what we would then comfortably call "cardiovascular disease."

Some might argue that cardiovascular disease is inevitable if you live long enough. Everyone's arteries and heart age and will eventually "wear out." That may be behind the perception that cancer is a lurking curse but heart disease is a natural occurrence. Yes, cardiovascular disease may be inevitable, just as every organ and joint will eventually fail. But the time frame is critical. If the aging process in your joints is destined not to produce disability until you are age one hundred, then joint replacement seems unnecessary. Similarly, if cardiovascular disease can be delayed in severity so that symptoms do not affect lifestyle until the age of one hundred, then I think we can conclude that we have effectively prevented heart disease, even if one-hundred-year-olds might disagree.

WHAT IS THE DISEASE OF THE ARTERIES CALLED?

There are a number of terms used to characterize the abnormalities of the artery wall that lead to illnesses that we call "cardiovascular disease." The original term is arteriosclerosis, which means that the large arteries, the ones you can see and feel, have become thickened and stiffened.[1] The lay term for this condition is "hardening of the arteries." A more recent term, atherosclerosis, implies that the wall of the artery has accumulated patches or plaques of cholesterol-containing material on the inner lining of the arteries. These can become obstructive to blood flow or they may fracture or rupture leading to clot formation—or thrombosis—in the artery that may suddenly obstruct blood flow. This scenario has led to use of a more contemporary term for the condition, atherothrombosis. It is a compound word invented to combine the description of the disease that leads to plaques with the process of clot formation that obstructs the artery and causes morbid events.

Arteriosclerosis and atherosclerosis or atherothrombosis often exist together. All progress with age, and some degree of the condition is probably inevitable if we live long enough. But the severity and rate of progression of these conditions are highly individual. Family history, and therefore inheritance, is a powerful predictor, but even in families with a high prevalence of premature disease, some descendants escape. All family members, of course, do not inherit the same genomic profile. Lifestyle (diet, exercise, smoking, etc.) may modify the rate of progression, but understanding the underlying biologic mechanisms that cause progression of the disease process has fueled the development of effective drug treatments that inhibit the process, regardless of the specific factors that may be accelerating it. So it really doesn't matter if one has inherited the tendency for the arteries to age or if one has carried on a lifestyle that encourages aging to be accelerated. Drugs that interfere with the biologic process of aging or arteriosclerosis or atherosclerosis can slow its progression.

LARGE ARTERIES VS. SMALL ARTERIES

There are two distinct kinds of arteries. The large arteries deliver the blood to the organs needing nourishment, and the small arteries distribute it within the tissue. The large arteries are often referred to as conduit arteries because they are like pipes that deliver water to the bathrooms of your house. But they aren't really like pipes because they are normally flexible so that their walls expand and contract with every heart beat. The pulse in these large arteries that you can feel in your neck, wrist, or groin results from the pressure rise with each heartbeat because your finger has compressed the flexible artery wall. When the artery is compressed, the next heartbeat generates a pressure wave that strikes your finger and would normally expand the artery. These conduit pipes or arteries don't produce much resistance to blood flow unless they get clogged up, thus requiring a visit from the plumber if it is a pipe in your home, or an interventional procedure by a cardiologist or surgeon if it's your cardio-vascular system. For many years, I was reluctant to use the plumbing analogy after seeing an elderly man who drank Drano in the hope that it would unclog his arteries.

The small arteries, on the other hand, are dynamic, microscopic tubes that profoundly influence the flow and distribution of blood flow in tissues.[2] This distribution of blood flow is critically important to organs like the kidney and brain. These small arteries can profoundly influence organ function. In a human brain, removed at autopsy, the brain tissue can be dissolved away chemically. What is left is a remarkably dense array of small arteries that occupy almost all the space you may have thought was occupied by brain tissue. The brain is really a gigantic array of small blood vessels. It's hardly surprising that disease of the small arteries can so influence the function of the brain and kidneys. This small artery disease probably represents the fundamental cause of most dementia and most kidney failure.

Changes in the artery wall that characterize arteriosclerosis or athero-sclerosis also occur in the small arteries. These small, microscopic arter-ies are especially sensitive to the influence of nitric oxide, a remarkable biologically active gas released from the inner lining of the arteries called the endothelium. A deficiency of nitric oxide—often referred to as endo-thelial dysfunction—leads to constriction and stiffening of these small arteries and to structural thickening of their walls. Although plaques do not form in these small arteries, the thickening itself can narrow the lumen or blood channel and result in some obstruction to tissue blood flow. These abnormalities of the small artery often precede and usually accompany the more visible changes in the large arteries identified as arteriosclerosis or atherosclerosis.

Another important factor in the artery wall disease is that narrowing and thickening of the small artery raises the vascular resistance to blood flow in the body and leads to a rise in blood pressure. Narrowing all the body's small arteries, like partial obstruction of the pipes in a plumbing system, always increases the force necessary to push fluid through the system. The pressure may rise only 5 or 10 mmHg, which means that an individual with a blood pressure of 100 mmHg might experience a rise to 110 mmHg, well within the normal range. But an individual whose blood pressure was normally 130 mmHg might develop so-called hypertensive blood pressures because of this change in the small artery wall. There-fore, the critical factor in defining small artery disease throughout the body may not be the absolute blood pressure but rather a subtle rise in pressure because of a rise in vascular resistance. These changes in the artery wall usually result from a deficiency of nitric oxide, and they usually progress over time unless treated.

Stiffening of the large arteries results in a rise in systolic blood pres-sure and usually a fall in diastolic pressure. That is the pattern well described with aging. That is why the definition of hypertension, which in the past focused on diastolic pressure, has gradually shifted to systolic pressure. Systolic pressure rises with age, so the elderly population has a very high incidence of hypertension, but the diastolic pressure tends to fall because the large arteries become more stiff.

PULSE WAVE VELOCITY

Most cardiologists and imaging specialists aren't much interested in the small arteries. They view the arteries as structures they can see on an angiogram and that they can fix with balloons, stents, or bypass grafts. When they hear about artery stiffness, they think of those large conduit arteries that run from the aorta to all the organs. The standard way to assess stiffness of these large arteries is by measuring the time, in microseconds, that it takes for the pulse wave, generated by pumping of the left ventricle, to travel from the beginning of the aorta, close to where the heart ejects the blood with each beat, to the arteries in the leg. The velocity of this pulse wave is directly related to the stiffness of the arteries.[3]

But when my associates and I think about artery stiffness, we consider separately this large artery stiffness and the stiffness of the small arteries, which can be detected by an effect on the oscillations in the pulse waveform induced by the small arteries.[4] This small artery stiffness, disregarded by most practitioners, may be the best early guide to artery wall disease because it provides an assessment of endothelial function or the adequacy of nitric oxide. How we assess that stiffness will be discussed in a later chapter.

FUNCTION OF THE HEART: PUMP, VALVES, AND RHYTHM

When experts think about heart disease, it is the heart's pumping function that draws most attention. We can appreciate each heartbeat if we feel the pulse in the wrist or neck, and we recognize that the heart is keeping us alive by pumping blood with each beat. I've had patients who have panicked because they thought their hearts had suddenly stopped because they were unable to feel their pulse or because they have experienced an extra or premature beat followed by a slight pause and then a jolt from an especially strong beat. Anxiety because you can't feel your pulse may be a neurotic reaction, but extra beats are a normal phenomenon in a world where almost nothing works perfectly all the time.

Disease of the heart ultimately affects its ability to deliver blood to the rest of the body. The most common cause in our society is disease of the coronary arteries nourishing the heart muscle. The heart muscle is normally in a fragile state of adequate nutrition. In contrast to all other organs, which are nourished by blood flowing in both systole (while the heart is beating) and diastole (between beats), the heart muscle must get all its blood supply in diastole. That's because in systole the contracting heart muscle squeezes shut all the blood vessels in the muscle so they cannot deliver blood to the working muscle. All the flow occurs in diastole, so even a modest deficiency of flow because of obstruction of the arteries can have serious consequences.

In addition to coronary artery obstruction, however, other disease may affect the heart's pumping ability. Viruses and toxins, such as alcohol, and nutritional deficiencies can lead to heart muscle disease called cardiomyopathy. Heart valve disease, either congenital or acquired, can progress to the point that it impairs the heart's ability to deliver blood to the tissues. All of these conditions can be recognized by structural changes in the heart long before symptoms develop. Most rhythm abnormalities are not lethal; extra beats and even bouts of fast and irregular rhythms are usually self-limiting and benign. When they are serious and life-threatening, however, they are always preceded by structural changes that can be recognized long before a lethal event can occur.

The structural change in the heart that predicts bad outcomes is a process called remodeling. What that means is the heart muscle cells—the myocytes—get bigger, and the supporting structure around the muscle cells grows and becomes stiffer. Like all muscles, the heart responds to an increased workload by an increase in mass of the muscle. A weight lifter exhibits the muscle mass changes in his chest and arms that result from the extra workload. Long-distance runners exhibit the heart muscle mass increase that reflects the extra burden placed on the heart. These normal growth processes are a form of muscular or cardiac remodeling. They are healthy, physiologic responses to workload. When the extra work is stopped, the tissues return to their normal state. The process is fully reversible.

Pathologic remodeling is a different process. In the heart, it is induced by some deficiency in heart function or structure that sets into motion growth processes designed to compensate for the impaired function. The heart muscle, or myocytes, grows in size, and collagen or scar tissue grows between the heart muscle cells. The process is not so easily reversible. The heart chamber often enlarges in a process called dilation.[5] The result of this slow and progressive process is a progressive loss of pumping power of the heart and a symptomatic condition called heart failure. This remodeling process can be recognized long before symptoms develop.

IS TREATMENT EFFECTIVE?

The presence of demonstrable disease in the artery wall or in the left ventricle in asymptomatic individuals has resulted in a real diagnostic dilemma. Should we identify it as a disease? Emphasis has been placed on treatment of acute symptoms of disease. We don't like to call it a disease until we get sick. Chest pain? Take an aspirin and call 911! Symptoms of stroke? Get immediately to the hospital. The health-care focus has been on management of the acute event and treatment to prevent its recurrence. The emphasis has not been on preventing the event in the first place, other than the usual public health recommendations to prevent obesity, avoid smoking, eat your fruits and vegetables, and exercise.

If treatment after the first symptoms were as effective as treatment before symptoms develop, then the current strategy would be appropriate. But it is not!

Once a coronary artery is blocked resulting in chest pain, heart muscle is permanently damaged and the coronary artery needs to be opened urgently by a catheterization technique or by surgery. The heart muscle damage, depending on its severity, may initiate a long-term progressive process in the heart that could eventually lead to heart failure or heart rhythm instability leading to sudden death. We have very effective treatments for all these chronic conditions, but it would be far better to prevent them instead of treating them. Effective drug therapy to slow vascular disease progression and to slow or block heart remodeling is currently available. I am confident even better and more focused therapy will become available in the future. The progressive process in diseased heart valves is not well enough understood to have resulted in an effective therapy to block it. Once again, however, if it is recognized as the priority it should be, new treatments will become available to block progressive valve distortion.

The brain damage from a stroke may be moderated by urgent surgery or by effective rehabilitation efforts, and we now may be able to reduce the risk of recurrent strokes. But long-term health is far better when a first stroke can be prevented.

Once a morbid event like a heart attack, stroke, or heart failure has occurred, life expectancy, and certainly life in good health, is shortened. The chance of living to one hundred is reduced. The question, then, is whether we can identify individuals with early disease likely to progress and initiate therapy that will halt or slow its progression. Whether we call it cardiovascular disease at this presymptomatic phase of the disease or whether we give it a different label is unimportant. We need to call it something, however, because we need to treat it. And we only treat things that are labeled!

MANAGEMENT VS. PREVENTION

Why has the health-care system placed more emphasis on management of the acute event rather than prevention of the acute event? The simplest answer is that the acute event gets the patient into the hands of the specialist where the newest technology can be applied. The health-care system thrives on expensive and effective management of such acute events. Hospitals, doctors, and device and drug manufacturers all profit from this management. And the management is remarkably effective. It is exciting health-care delivery.

The party line is that the health-care system does emphasize prevention. The message comes from the American Heart Association and your local and regional health departments. Prevent heart attacks and strokes by reducing your risk factors. Lose weight, exercise, reduce your consumption of red meats, eat fish. The media would lead you to think that cardiovascular disease is self-inflicted. All you need to do is change your lifestyle and those nasty heart attacks and strokes won't occur.

These messages from professional health-care organizations adhere to the traditional distinction between what is called primary and secondary prevention. The terminology appeared before we had developed the ability to identify and track disease progression. Secondary prevention was defined as the attempt to prevent recurrent events, such as a second heart attack or a second stroke. The assumption was that in the absence of a symptomatic event, the patient was healthy and all efforts at prevention should be labeled "primary prevention." The view has been that it is difficult to justify initiating treatment in these healthy people, so the emphasis should be on lifestyle changes to control risk factors. On the other hand, secondary prevention—after an event has already occurred—should include aggressive treatment. After all, we know these people have disease that needs treatment.

But what if we know disease is progressing even if the individual has not sustained a symptomatic event? More than half the adult American population will suffer a cardiovascular morbid event before the age of one hundred.[6] Wouldn't it be appropriate to initiate treatment in those individuals in an attempt to prevent a first event? Should we call that primary prevention? Or should we call that secondary prevention because we can find early disease and we want to slow its progression? Or better still, why call it prevention? It is actually treatment, not prevention. It is treatment of early disease to slow its progression. The long-term goal certainly is to prevent future morbid events, but the management is aimed at slowing progression of disease.

The health-care establishment and media emphasis on risk factor control for primary prevention of morbid events disregards our ability to detect and track disease. Cancer management doesn't emphasize risk factor intervention as much as they do early detection. Mammograms and colonoscopies are not restricted to those with risk factors but are rather recommended for everyone to detect early disease. Why doesn't the health-care system also recommend detection of early cardiovascular disease as a strategy to identify the need for intervention? Medicare doesn't reimburse for any test aimed at evaluating cardiovascular health in an asymptomatic patient. But removing a malignant polyp from the colon is not considered primary prevention and it is richly rewarded by Medicare. It is treatment of a disease detected only by colonoscopy, and the colonoscopy is justified by the fact that it may find disease that needs to be treated.

There also may be an economic incentive for the difference in strategy between cardiovascular disease and cancer management. Detection of early cancer leads to surgical intervention to remove it. The process both generates revenue and appears definitive. Everybody wins. On the other hand, detection of early cardiovascular disease should ideally elicit a prescription for drugs. There is little revenue for the doctor, none for the hospital, and little for the pharmaceutical industry because all the effective drugs are generic and cheap. The public is suspicious of prescription drugs and skeptical of their benefit in people who do not think they are sick. It isn't a dramatic enough finding, like a polyp in the colon, to instill concern in the lay community that something must be done. There has been no lobbying to change the public's behavior or health insurance policies.

There may be another reason for health-care skepticism of early disease detection. The statistical association of risk factors with future morbid events, first documented in the Framingham study (a population study that has been tracking people in Framingham, Massachusetts, for at least two generations), has led to a number of algorithms or formulae that claim to calculate an individual's risk, based largely on the assessment of these risk factors, which include age and gender.[7] Age, in fact, not surprisingly becomes the major contributor to risk calculation. When dealing with a large population of people aged twenty to ninety, it is hardly unexpected that age will be a powerful driver of risk for cardiovascular disease. The promoters of these algorithms have discounted the value of newer measures of risk, including early disease markers, by noting that the addition of these measures do not appear to improve the predictive accuracy of the algorithms. That has also led guideline developers to discourage use of early disease markers in routine patient assessment.

The effort to document the value of early detection has been flawed by the methodology used. In most instances a single test has been used, and often this test is an imaging assessment for advanced disease in a single site. For example, X-ray assessment of coronary calcium provides a definite marker for atherosclerosis in a coronary artery. Then why doesn't it improve the discriminatory value of the algorithm in predicting who will have a future heart attack? The reason may be that people younger than fifty don't have calcium in their coronary arteries, even if they have atherosclerotic plaques. Younger people have coronary disease that has not yet calcified, a process that is age-dependent. And age is already in all the algorithms as a powerful risk factor. Age as a population risk, unrelated to the individual's biologic state, may reduce the discriminatory value of calcium if that is the sole test being performed. So single imaging tests may lack the sensitivity (finding disease if it is present) to improve the algorithms based on risk factors. Furthermore, expert panels express concern that imaging tests often detect abnormalities that lead specialists to intervene surgically when the detected lesions are asymptomatic and should not be treated. Similar skepticism has grown recently regarding the benefits of the search for cancers using mammograms and prostate blood test screening. The invasive procedures used in response to the screening may produce more harm than good.

More comprehensive assessment of early cardiovascular disease using a number of tests has been our strategy. This method identifies early disease in many individuals who are deemed low-risk by the Framingham and other risk algorithms.

CAN EARLY CARDIOVASCULAR DISEASE BE DETECTED?

Newer technology and better application of older technology now make it possible to rather simply and noninvasively study the function and structure of the arteries and the heart, the two organs that account for all cardiovascular disease. Individuals destined to have heart attacks, strokes, and other cardiovascular diseases always exhibit abnormalities of the arteries or heart long before they become symptomatic. Individuals without such abnormalities cannot suffer from these life-threatening events. These acute events are the consequence of progression of the abnormalities detected by the study of function and structure of the arteries and heart.

In the old days, until at least the 1980s, there was little incentive to find out if one had disease in the arteries or heart. If one had no symptoms that were impairing quality of life, there was no reason to search for early disease. We had developed effective treatments to relieve people who were sick, but we had no evidence that we could alter the course of asymptomatic people with early disease. But clinical trials carried out in the past thirty years now make it clear that treatment to slow progression of early disease can effectively prevent those acute events from occurring, and the earlier one identifies the abnormalities the more effective the therapy should be.[8]

The response of some in the medical establishment to our promotion of early detection for targeted treatment is to dismiss it as unnecessary and too expensive. They often claim that the current emphasis on risk factor detection and reduction is adequate for identification and treatment to prevent heart attacks and strokes. They will also state that the testing we utilize to evaluate the structure and function of the cardiovascular system is needlessly complicated and expensive. They are wrong on both counts. The current approach recommended for evaluation—risk factor assessment and targeted treatment—misses the majority of individuals destined to have heart attacks and strokes. It does identify an advanced disease subgroup with high blood pressure, diabetes, and very high cholesterol levels, but these high-risk individuals represent only a small fraction of people having heart attacks and strokes every year. A focus on risk algorithms may successfully identify the "low-hanging fruit" of advanced disease, but it misses the majority of those who are going to suffer from cardiovascular disease, perhaps not in five or ten years but in twenty or thirty years. Detecting the disease early and slowing its progression is the best preventive strategy. The trouble and cost of doing the testing are dwarfed by the costs and trouble of doing mammograms and colonoscopies whose long-term benefit is controversial but whose performance is widely recommended.

Subsequent chapters will explore in more detail how the current emphasis on risk factors is leaving most of the at-risk population unprotected and needlessly imposing interventions on others not at risk.

CONTEMPORARY UNDERSTANDING

- Heart attacks and strokes are complications of advancing disease in the arteries. If the early disease is identified, such events are not "unpredictable." Indeed, treatment will slow progression and delay or prevent such events from occurring during one's optimal life expectancy.
- Heart attacks, strokes, and diabetes are largely the result of inherited disease factors. Lifestyle may alter the rate of the disease's progression, but its impact is only modest. Drug therapy, however, may have a profound effect in slowing progression, regardless of what is stimulating the process.
- Sudden death is almost always predictable because of the presence of early structural changes in the heart. Therapy may be effective in preventing it, particularly implanted defibrillators.
- Impaired circulation to the legs is the result of progressive disease in the arteries supplying the legs with blood supply. These arteries are more likely to develop blockages with age, but it is a consequence of

artery wall disease (arteriosclerosis, atherosclerosis) that can be identified and treated long before symptoms develop.

- Kidney disease and dementia are usually cardiovascular diseases because the most common cause is obstruction of blood flow in the small arteries nourishing the tissues. Early recognition can lead to treatment to slow its progression.

2

MYOCARDIAL INFARCTION OR HEART ATTACK

CONVENTIONAL WISDOM

- Myocardial infarction, or heart attack, is a sudden and usually painful event in which the heart muscle is damaged because of a lack of adequate blood flow to nourish the tissue.
- Myocardial infarctions are often brought on by stress.
- Heart attacks are often the result of a long-term unhealthy lifestyle.
- Myocardial infarctions are often fatal.
- They usually occur without warning and can't be predicted.
- Severe chest pain and sweating are characteristic of the episode.
- Men are far more likely to have a myocardial infarction than women.

WHAT IS A HEART ATTACK?

The phrase "heart attack" is a lay term that has no medical meaning. It usually refers to an acute myocardial infarction (or AMI) that presents, often in a previously apparently healthy individual, with crushing chest pain that may radiate to the left arm or jaw and is associated with weakness and sweating. An electrocardiogram (ECG), usually recorded by emergency medics, will show the telltale signs of an AMI with acute changes in the electrical signal from the heart characterized by elevation of the junction between the QRS complex and the subsequent T-wave.

The QRS describes the electrical signal leading to contraction of the pumping chamber, and the T-wave describes the signal during the mechanical recovery period between beats.

But all heart attacks or myocardial infarctions don't present the same way, and all are not equal. We now define a myocardial infarction as the sudden destruction of heart muscle cells by insufficient nourishing blood flow. We now have a sensitive means of detecting destruction of heart muscle cells by measuring an enzyme in blood released from heart cells that are irreparably injured. The newest enzyme test, a high-sensitivity method for detecting troponin, is so sensitive that some feel it might end up finding heart muscle damage when it hasn't really occurred. Nonetheless, an elevation of one of these cardiac enzymes has become a critical component of the diagnosis of myocardial infarction. A stab wound in the chest or even blunt trauma from a steering wheel in a car accident can damage or destroy heart muscle cells, and some viruses can attack and damage heart cells. In these conditions, enzyme levels in the blood may be elevated, but the elevation is not attributed to a myocardial infarction. An infarction is diagnosed when other such causes are excluded and the muscle damage can be attributed to a sudden inadequacy of coronary blood flow to nourish the muscle. The ECG changes may be diagnostic, especially if they evolve over time, but uncertainty often persists. Most emergency rooms have developed protocols to observe questionable cases until there is diagnostic certainty.

TWO KINDS OF HEART ATTACKS

We now know there are two distinct kinds of myocardial infarctions—the classical kind, described above, and a more subtle form that has become more common in recent years. The first, the classical one with crushing chest pain, is caused almost invariably by a sudden clot in a major coronary artery. If the electrocardiogram (ECG) reveals the tell-tale sign of this problem—an elevated ST segment—the patient is usually rushed to the catheterization laboratory where the clot in the artery is visualized, the artery opened by inflation of a balloon to squash the clot against the artery wall, and the opening maintained with a plastic stent placed through the catheter. This is a STEMI, or ST-elevation myocardial infarction.

If the above procedure is performed soon enough after the clot has formed, damage to the heart muscle from the clot can be minimized.[1] The sooner the artery can be opened, the less the damage to heart muscle. That is why hospitals are graded these days on their "door-to-balloon" or "door-to-needle" time,[2] with a goal of getting appropriate patients from the emergency room to the catheterization lab in less than ninety minutes or even in less than an hour. Of course, the biggest obstacle is the delay between the onset of pain and arrival at the hospital. That's where education and emergency services come in.

The other kind of heart attack is not caused by a clot and does not result in an elevated ST segment on the ECG. But it is caused by a sustained insufficiency of blood supply to meet the needs of the heart muscle. It occurs in individuals with severe disease in their coronary arteries, either plaques in the large arteries that partially obstruct blood flow or structural narrowing of the small arteries that are not visualized on an angiogram. There is no sudden obstruction by a clot. The damage from inadequate blood supply often occurs predominantly in the inner layers of the heart muscle, thus the older term "subendocardial myocardial infarction," meaning the inner layer of the heart muscle. The damaged heart muscle releases enzymes like troponin, but usually less than in a "STEMI."[3] Nonetheless, the diagnosis of myocardial infarction is made, but a rush to the cath lab is not appropriate. These patients may ultimately benefit from opening the chronic and partially obstructed arteries or bypass surgery to restore better perfusion, but these procedures are designed to prevent future events, not to alter the degree of damage from the current event. The important thing to know is that STEMIs can occur in patients with only mild underlying coronary artery disease, but non-STEMIs generally occur in people with advanced disease in whom the long-term prognosis may not be good. Both are the result of plaque build-up in the coronary arteries, a process that can now be prevented. But STEMIs are precipitated by a clot and non-STEMIs by demand for blood flow not adequately met by the chronically narrowed coronary arteries.

WHAT ARE THE COMPLICATIONS OF MYOCARDIAL INFARCTION?

Infarction or damage to heart muscle cells is a serious event. Until the 1960s, acute heart attacks killed thousands of individuals before they could get to a hospital. The mortality rate even in those who reached the hospital was about 20 percent.[4] Hospitalization lasted for weeks because there was no other therapy, and the goal was to protect the patient while the injured heart muscle was healing.

All that has now changed. We have a 911 phone system that should quickly reach urban dwellers with emergency services and transport. We have drugs to dissolve clots and prevent new ones from forming. We have drugs and devices that can support function of the impaired pumping chamber and treat what would otherwise be heart failure. We have electrical devices that can protect against heart rhythm disturbances, which are another complication of myocardial infarction. More patients now reach the hospital, including those who previously died on the street or at home, and the in-hospital mortality rate after an acute myocardial infarction is now well below 5 percent.[5] Hospitalizations have now usually been reduced to only a few days.

But that doesn't mean heart attacks are now only a "bump in the road" of life. If heart muscle is damaged, there is always the potential for more future damage. And if heart muscle damage is extensive enough, the heart may undergo a condition called structural "remodeling," a molecular and cellular process in which the remaining cells enlarge and alter their shape.[6] The long-term result of this "remodeling" is a change in the geometry of the heart chamber, which impairs its function as a pump. Heart failure may ensue, even years after the initial damage to the heart muscle, and rhythm disturbances leading to sudden death can also occur. So a heart attack is a major event that is far better to have prevented than to treat.

ARE HEART ATTACKS PREDICTABLE?

The answer to that question is complicated. Yes, we should be able to determine who is at risk. But no, we can't really tell if an event will occur, and we certainly can't predict when such an event will occur.

Myocardial infarction does not occur in individuals without athero-sclerosis in their coronary arteries. Does everyone have such disease? Although the medical world was taken aback by the documentation by autopsy of coronary disease in many young soldiers killed in the Korean War,[7] severe or obstructive disease was not common. It is true that the disease starts early when it is inherited in the genetic code. But the vast majority of young people do not have advanced disease. With aging more disease occurs, but the severity of disease varies greatly from individual to individual. Furthermore, these visual assessments of disease severity disregard the small, invisible coronary arteries that contribute importantly to inadequate blood supply in many individuals, particularly women.

How can we determine who is at risk? Atherosclerosis is a systemic disease not localized to the coronary arteries. By studying structure and function of more accessible arteries, it is possible to establish the general health of the small and large arteries. If they are abnormal, it is likely the coronaries are also abnormal, or at least may become abnormal. These individuals are at risk. In the absence of disease in these other arteries, it is highly unlikely that a heart attack will occur. Of course artery health is a dynamic process. It may change with time, so continued surveillance is critical. The process of assessing artery health will be considered in a later chapter.

Even if we can identify who is at risk because of the presence of atherosclerosis, why do heart attacks occur when they do? What precipi-tates the acute event? The presence of atherosclerosis in the coronary artery, however it is identified, does not divulge if and when a myocardial infarction will occur. There are clearly other factors at work. The most important may be the tendency for blood to form a small clot on the cholesterol-containing plaque on the wall of a coronary artery. That ten-dency may be enhanced by sudden change in the plaque itself or in the platelets, the small particles in blood that instigate the clotting process. Aspirin may reduce the risk of the platelets sticking together to form a clot.

When the plaque cracks or ruptures, it exposes various cellular and inflammatory substances that encourage a clot to form.[8] Plaque cracking or rupture may be induced by physical activities, such as an intense activity like shoveling snow. When platelets are in some way activated, perhaps even by emotional stresses and hormone release, they have a greater likelihood of instigating a clot on a cracked plaque.

Anecdotes abound regarding individuals who have dropped dead or sustained heart attacks in the setting of what is described as emotional stress. It could reflect rupture of a plaque or a change in platelet "stickiness." But these anecdotes are difficult to trust. We need to know more about the individual and the event. Some such episodes may be cases of what is now called Takatsubo syndrome, a more descriptive term being "Broken Heart Syndrome."[9] This condition is named after the Japanese octopus pot because that is the shape the patient's left ventricle or pumping chamber takes on during the attack. The event is clearly induced by emotional stress and is not caused by an abnormality of the coronary artery. It acutely impairs the pumping ability of the heart and certainly mimics a myocardial infarction, but it is fully reversible and leaves no deformity or disability. Unfortunately, myocardial infarctions do both.

So, although we aren't good at predicting when a myocardial infarction will occur, we usually should be able to predict well enough who is at risk to confine our preventive efforts to those with unhealthy arteries, or early disease, likely to progress. That is not what is being done today. By focusing our attention on individuals with high so-called risk factors, such as blood pressure and cholesterol levels, and not on identifying unhealthy arteries, we are missing the majority of individuals at risk for heart attacks. That is a deficiency in our health-care system that can be corrected.

But there also may be a certain degree of bad luck involved that we cannot control. I remember a young man brought into our emergency room a number of years ago on life support. He had had a cardiac arrest in a restaurant and was resuscitated by the medics who rushed to his side. He didn't survive. On autopsy he had a single plaque at the origin of his left anterior descending coronary artery, the one nourishing the whole front wall of his heart. A clot had formed on this plaque and obstructed the artery. The rest of his coronary arteries appeared to be entirely normal. I'm not certain if he had generalized disease that we could have detected, but certainly the single plaque and its dangerous location could only be attributed to bad luck. It was like stopping for a cup of coffee in the World Trade Center on the morning of September 11, 2001.

HOW DO HEART ATTACKS RELATE TO OTHER CARDIOVASCULAR MORBID EVENTS?

Although heart attacks are the most high-profile acute cardiovascular event, the same disease process that affects coronary arteries (atherosclerosis) coexists in all the arteries of the body, especially in the arteries to the brain, the legs, and the kidneys. Obstruction of blood flow to the brain results in an acute neurological deficit, from a transient loss of speech or motor function to a permanent paralysis of up to 50 percent of the body. Obstruction of blood flow to the legs results in pain, pallor, and coolness in an extremity. In the kidney, the process is usually more gradual with a decrease in kidney function that can only be documented by the accumulation in the body of waste products usually excreted in the urine.

It is hardly surprising that the presence of disease in any one of these vascular beds increases the likelihood of disease developing in one of the other vascular beds. This disease coexists in the heart, brain, legs, and kidneys. But there are subtle differences in the atherosclerotic process in these various organs. In the coronary bed, most of the symptomatic disease comes from obstruction of the large arteries visualized by angiograms. Even here, however, some individuals, more often women, are more likely to suffer from small artery disease not visualized by angiograms.[10] In the brain, large artery disease usually causes strokes, but small artery disease contributes to memory loss and dementia. In the kidney, it is largely the small arteries that contribute to kidney failure. And in the legs, both large arteries and small arteries are important contributors to the disease called peripheral vascular disease. The process in the arteries is similar in all the organs, but why some individuals develop more disease in one organ than another remains a mystery.

Although some may be fatalistic about this disease and claim that it is an inevitable complication of aging, I disagree. The atherosclerotic process may progress over time in everyone, but its severity and rate of progression are very individualized. If your parents and grandparents had strokes or heart attacks, you are at a statistically higher risk from an inheritance standpoint, but whether you have individually inherited this tendency is a chance phenomenon ruled by the X or Y genes you have acquired. Whether you do or do not have progressive disease can only be determined by assessing the function and structure of your arteries. If disease is present, it can be accelerated by poor lifestyle choices, such as an imprudent diet, obesity, smoking, and lack of exercise. If it's not present, then these lifestyle choices are less important. But truly slowing or halting the disease from progressing requires drug therapy, which will be discussed later. Lifestyle changes alone are unlikely to have a profound effect on disease progression.

The goal: Identify and treat early disease before heart attacks and strokes occur!

CONTEMPORARY UNDERSTANDING

- Heart attacks and other cardiovascular morbid events are usually a complication of underlying atherosclerotic disease of the large or small arteries.
- Morbid events are as common in women as in men, but they may present differently because of a difference in the severity of small and large artery disease.
- The acute events warrant urgent efforts to restore obstructed or deficient blood flow.
- Modern procedure and device therapy can reduce the severity and complication rate of these acute events.
- The most effective therapy would be to recognize as early as possible the underlying disease likely to cause such events and to intervene to slow its progression or to cause its regression.

3

BLOOD PRESSURE

CONVENTIONAL WISDOM

- Blood pressure in the hypertensive range is an important risk factor for heart attacks and strokes.
- A blood pressure less than 140/90 mmHg, especially if your cholesterol is within the normal range, indicates you are safe from cardiovascular disease.
- Administration of antihypertensive drugs is appropriate therapy for patients with blood pressures in the hypertensive range.
- Lifestyle changes that reduce blood pressure to below the hypertensive threshold make it unnecessary to take drugs.
- The treatment goal in hypertension is to lower blood pressure, regardless of how it is accomplished.

HOW BLOOD PRESSURE IS MEASURED

Blood pressure measurement with a cuff placed around the upper arm is so simple that it is incorporated into almost all medical visits and evaluations. Instruments are routinely available in drug stores and health clubs for self-measurement. Along with body weight, temperature, and pulse rate, blood pressure measurement constitutes the standard assessment of the health of an individual. When doctors see patients in their office or clinic, these measurements, usually performed by a nurse or an aide, already appear on the paper chart or electronic record before the doctor steps into the room. The rationale for this tradition may relate more to the ease of data collection than to the importance of the information.

This approach to medical care was of course not always practiced. Until the 1900s, there was no technique available to measure the pressure of the blood in the arteries. When a practical method became available, some physicians criticized its use because it might dissuade doctors from what was then the tradition of careful palpation of the arteries at various sites in the body to assess the characteristics of the pulse. With experience, these diagnosticians believed they could determine the health of the underlying arteries. They were concerned that a measurement of blood pressure using these new devices would be a simple tool that would be less informative than their educated fingers. I'm not sure they were entirely wrong.

The blood pressure is the pressure generated by the force of the heart's contraction into a closed system; that is, all the arteries that branch from the aorta that receives the blood ejected by each beat of the heart. The force that the heart must generate to eject that blood is influenced by the resistance or oppositional force imposed by the arteries in that closed system. So the pressure in the arteries is determined primarily by the interaction of the amount of blood pumped by the heart, the rate at which it is ejected with each contraction of the left ventricle, and the resistance imposed by the arteries into which the blood is ejected. This resistance is largely determined by the structure of the arteries and their functional state; that is, whether they are constricted or stiff rather than flexible and relaxed.

The absolute level of that pressure was unknown until Reverend Stephen Hales from Cambridge, England, placed a small-bore brass pipe into the neck artery of a mare in 1733.[1] He measured the pressure by attaching his metal tube to a 9-foot-long glass tube that he mounted vertically above the animal. He observed how high the column of blood rose in the tube before equilibrating. He measured the height as 8 feet 3 inches or 246 centimeters. The impracticality of using a column of blood or, similarly, a column of water to determine the pressure in the arteries is apparent from the height of the tubing required by Hales.

After Hales's experiment, it became clear that an alternative device was needed to measure arterial pressure. It was the Frenchman Poiseuille who developed the mercury manometer in 1828. Since mercury, or Hg, is

13.6 times heavier than water or blood, the arterial pressure will support a column of mercury 1/13.6 times as high as the blood column. Hales's experiments would have been much easier had he used a column of mercury instead of a column of blood. Hales's mare's blood pressure would have supported a column of mercury only 7 inches high, which is equivalent to 180 mm of mercury, the apparent pressure of that poor befuddled and apprehensive horse. Since Poiseuille, it has become conventional to report all pressures in mmHg, even though environmentally dangerous mercury has now largely been eliminated from medical care facilities.

Having a mercury column to support the pressure of blood coming from puncturing an artery is certainly not a feasible way to measure the pressure in healthy patients. The routine clinical measurement of blood pressure did not become available until the work of Von Basch, Riva-Rocci, and Korotkoff had demonstrated the use of an air-filled cuff surrounding the upper arm and a stethoscope placed over the brachial artery at the crease of the elbow.[2] The goal was to hear the sounds generated by the gush of blood into the artery when the cuff pressure constricting the arm is reduced to below the systolic pressure (the pressure when the heart is contracting). These sounds disappear when the pressure in the cuff is reduced to below the diastolic pressure (the pressure before the next heartbeat) and the artery is no longer even momentarily occluded. For more than one hundred years, this has been the standard method for measuring blood pressure. It has been modified in recent years by automated techniques that eliminate the stethoscope and make self-measurement simple, but the concept of assessing the pressure by determining how much pressure must be added to the cuff to occlude the artery has not changed. It is an indirect technique because rather than measuring pressure directly from the artery, it depends on the compressive force of the air in the cuff around the arm. The assumption is that when the pressure in the cuff surrounding the artery is effective in occluding the artery, the pressure in the cuff has surpassed the pressure in the artery. The accuracy of this indirect measurement may be influenced by such things as arm fat, arm shape, and cuff width.

In my early days as an inquisitive clinical scientist, I remember a young patient with a very fat and tapering upper arm. His cuff blood pressure was very elevated, and he was being treated by his physician with drugs to lower it. He was not responding to treatment and was referred to me for help with his management. I was so troubled by the cuff measurements that I convinced him to accept a needle in his artery to allow us to measure the pressure directly. His pressure was normal, and the drugs were stopped. I never had a follow-up on the patient, so I can only hope that my unusual procedure served him well.

Despite these potential errors in indirect measurement of pressure, the cuff measurement has brought pressure measurement into routine practice and has certainly spawned a generation of attention to pressure and its treatment. It also has reduced the doctor's interest in feeling the arteries in an attempt to assess their health.

WHY BLOOD PRESSURE IS IMPORTANT

The ability to measure blood pressure in clinical practice was not immediately matched by the ability to properly utilize the data. Blood pressure varies quite widely from individual to individual. It's not like body temperature, which is rather tightly controlled. Temperatures above 98.6 degrees are pretty reliably abnormal, and they don't vary that much from day to day or during the day. Indeed, women may use very small daily changes of less than one degree to track their time of monthly ovulation. In contrast, blood pressure bounces around from day to day, varies throughout the day in a fairly predictable way (lower at night, higher in the morning), and is influenced by exercise and stress. This variability has always complicated the interpretation of the health implications of a blood pressure measurement. Because of the recognition of the influence of exercise and stress, it was deemed from the early days that in order to characterize an individual's blood pressure, it should be measured when the patient is comfortably seated and at rest. The patient's emotional state, of course, could not be controlled.

The individual variability of blood pressure has always raised the issue of how much of that variability might be inherited, or genetic, and how much is environmental. Probably the best experimental data to address that issue came from a remarkable study carried out at the University of Minnesota several decades ago. The investigators identified a substantial group of identical twins who were separated at birth and raised independently, usually unaware of the existence of the twin. Even though their environmental conditions and upbringing varied widely, their blood pressures were remarkably similar. Since the genetics of these identical twins were identical, it was clear that heredity was a powerful determinant of their blood pressure. We now also know that hypertension, that condition associated with blood pressures well above any normal range, often runs in families and therefore is assumed to be at least in part inherited.

The ability to measure blood pressure led to the recognition that very high levels, observed in only a small fraction of people, were associated with heart attacks, strokes, heart failure, and death. This condition was called hypertension, and the level of blood pressure that qualified for the diagnosis was set in the mid-twentieth century at about 160/100 mmHg. That means that when the heart pumped, the cuff pressure needed to occlude the artery in the arm was 160 mmHg (the systolic pressure), and when the heart was resting before the next beat, the pressure needed to occlude the artery was 100 mmHg (the diastolic pressure). Drugs to safely lower blood pressure were not available in those days, and there was no consensus that lowering the blood pressure was a prudent thing to do. Many experts claimed the elevated blood pressure represented nature's way of forcing enough blood through constricted blood vessels and that efforts to lower it would be dangerous.

It was not until the 1960s that carefully designed trials compared placebo or dummy pill therapy with safe blood-pressure-lowering drug therapy in hypertensive patients. These studies showed that the drugs that lower blood pressure produce dramatic protection from strokes, heart failure, and death, although the incidence of heart attacks was troublingly not affected.[3] The previously skeptical medical community began to embrace antihypertensive drug therapy. Along with this new evidence for the benefit of blood-pressure lowering came an appreciation that maybe 160/100 mmHg was too stringent a criterion for the diagnosis of hypertension. The threshold for the diagnosis, but not necessarily the threshold for treatment, gradually settled on 140/90 mmHg.

The issue of which is more important, the systolic pressure or the diastolic pressure, has also gone through several generations of debate. The early feeling was that the diastolic pressure is a better measure of the "tone" of the arteries and a better guide to the presence of hypertension. Indeed, a diastolic pressure of 90 mmHg or higher was generally accepted as the diagnostic criterion for hypertension. But epidemiological data demonstrated that with normal aging, the diastolic pressure falls and the systolic pressure rises as a consequence of stiffening of the large arteries. [4] Therefore, in individuals over the age of sixty, the systolic pressure serves as a better guide to the presence of hypertension. The current guidelines identify both. So hypertension is defined as a condition in which either the systolic pressure is at least 140 mmHg or the diastolic pressure is at least 90 mmHg.

Age is of course a major confounding variable. In our society, as noted above, systolic blood pressure rises with age, probably because the arteries become more rigid and thus oppose the force of the blood ejected from the heart. That may not necessarily be true in less-developed societies or those with different genetic characteristics. A flexible or distensible artery will expand when confronted with the blood ejected by a heartbeat. The rigid artery resists expansion, and this leads to a greater pressure rise. In the old days, people were taught that a normal upper level of systolic blood pressure is 100 mmHg plus your age. Guidelines long ago abandoned that idea, particularly because a large trial showed that lowering this age-related high systolic blood pressure with drugs resulted in a reduced risk of cardiovascular morbid events. [5] Recommended levels to define normal and abnormal blood pressures are now independent of age. That, of course, means that as people age, they are more and more likely to become hypertensive.

Choosing a threshold level for the diagnosis of hypertension has always been an arbitrary process. When large databases of blood pressure values became available, especially in carefully selected populations, epidemiologists explored the implications. They found a relationship between the recorded level of the resting blood pressure and the future risk of heart attacks, strokes, heart failure, and death. That relationship was strikingly linear. That is, every increment in blood pressure in the population was associated with an increment in risk of death from cardiovascular disease, whether it was an increase in systolic pressure from 140 to 150 mmHg or an increase in diastolic pressure from 100 to 110 mmHg. [6] There was no magic threshold above which morbid events occurred and below which there were no morbid events.

That is the strength, and weakness, of population data. There is great strength in numbers. The data I refer to were collected in hundreds of thousands of patients. It takes numbers that large to obtain statistically reliable and reproducible data on future morbid events that can be related back to the initial blood pressure recordings. But how do these population data relate to individual patients, particularly using a measurement that is so variable in such individuals? And how predictive really is the pressure measurement? Yes, there is an incremental risk in the population, but the magnitude of that risk increase is remarkably small, possibly 5 or 10 percent for a 10 mmHg rise in pressure. That increment is highly statistically significant, which means we can reliably conclude that it is a real association, not a statistical fluke. But is it meaningful for an individual to know that his risk of dying from a heart attack or stroke is, for example, 1 in 5 versus 1 in 5.5?

So how did the medical establishment decide that 140/90 mmHg should be the threshold for the diagnosis of hypertension? It was largely an arbitrary decision based on the desire not to capture too many otherwise healthy people into the diagnostic category but to include those who on the basis of their higher pressures belonged to a population of individuals at higher risk. There was and still is no other diagnostic technique recommended to identify the disease category "hypertension." It's based entirely on resting blood pressure, and that's all!

Since so-called resting blood pressure may vary considerably from moment to moment, health-care providers were saddled with the responsibility of using a continuously variable measurement to place individuals into a lifelong disease category, one that could have great implications for their life insurance rates and their health-care costs. Furthermore, the measurement itself was dependent on how the cuff was applied to the arm and how well the nurse or physician examiner could discern the sounds emanating from the artery, or the accuracy of the algorithm contained in electronic devices programmed to identify the systolic and diastolic pressures. The medical establishment was well aware of these weaknesses of the diagnostic criteria. They resolved it, they thought, by telling health-care providers to take the pressure several times and average the results. When there was uncertainty, they advised, bring the patient back for several subsequent visits and average all the readings. Or better still, have the patient measure his or her blood pressure at home or provide him or her with an ambulatory monitor that can be worn over a period of days to record the pressure at regular intervals. The diagnosis inevitably became a game of numbers, and how providers were to use these home or ambulatory pressures to plan management has never been clearly defined.

Patients don't like to be told they have a disease. An elevated office blood pressure, they often claim, is because of stress in their office or difficulty finding a parking place. Physicians are similarly loath to tell their patients there is something wrong with them, especially if it means they must start them on lifelong drug therapy. These are disincentives for the diagnosis and treatment of an elevated blood pressure and for the diagnosis of "hypertension."

In recent years, hypertension experts became concerned with the rigid and unrealistic threshold for the diagnosis of hypertension. They were further influenced by the growing evidence, first documented by data from the long-standing Framingham study in Massachusetts, that people with blood pressures over 120/80 mmHg but less than 140/90 mmHg have more cardiovascular morbid events than those with blood pressures less than 120/80 mmHg.[7] These observations are of course entirely consistent with the idea that blood pressure and risk are associated on a continuous basis, not exclusively by a threshold.

In order to be consistent with the data, they decided to label those with blood pressures between 120–139/80–89 mmHg with a diagnosis. It couldn't be "hypertension" because they were not going to advocate treatment. But they wanted the patients and doctors to know they were at higher risk. They agreed on the term "pre-hypertension."[8] It may not have been a wise choice. The term implies that if we wait long enough, these individuals will become hypertensive, that is, their blood pressures will rise to greater than 140/90 mmHg. In some patients it may, but many of these individuals suffer morbid events when their blood pressure is still below 140/90 mmHg. Nonetheless, the "pre-hypertension" category provided doctors, if they chose to use it, a new diagnostic term in which to pigeonhole their patients. It didn't resolve the problem of variability in technique or in pressure itself. It put the patients on a "watch list" but nothing more.

WHY BLOOD PRESSURE IS ASSOCIATED WITH RISK

Patients rarely die or become disabled these days as a direct result of an elevated blood pressure. Modest elevation of blood pressure, which is the usual current form of the disease, does not in itself usually cause morbid events, such as heart attacks and strokes. These events are the consequence of damage to the arteries, usually sustained over long periods of time, and it is this damage that may be accelerated when the blood pressure is elevated.

It is important to understand the difference in pressure effects on the cerebral arteries, which cause strokes, and the coronary arteries, which cause myocardial infarction or heart attacks. The cerebral arteries are subjected to the systolic blood pressure that is measured by the arm cuff. These arteries may be fragile. Very high pressures can damage or rupture them. There is consequently a powerful relationship between strokes and very high blood pressures.

The coronary arteries, on the other hand, are not exposed to that systolic pressure. During systole, when the heart is contracting, the coronary arteries are squeezed shut by the contracting heart muscle. Blood does not flow into these arteries during systole, but its perfusion occurs entirely in diastole when the pressure is low. Thus high blood pressure has little influence on the walls of the coronary arteries, although it certainly places an extra workload on the heart muscle that must contract against the systolic pressure. These are the reasons that heart failure is a common complication of hypertension and its incidence is greatly reduced by all drugs that lower blood pressure, whereas heart attack incidence and response to treatment is more controversial.

The disease "hypertension" has changed over the years. Until drug therapy for hypertension became widely used in the 1960s, the disease often appeared in a severe form. It was not unusual to see individuals with pressures as high as 220/120 mmHg admitted to the hospital suffering from the consequence of their high pressure. They might have been short of breath because of failure of the heart to empty adequately under the burden of the very high resistance. They might have experienced a stroke due to bleeding into the brain caused by the high pressure rupturing an artery. They might have had severe headache and confusion due to swelling of the brain resulting from the high pressures in the brain arteries. They sometimes had a condition we call "malignant hypertension," not because it was related to cancer but because it was associated with severe damage to the arteries that could lead to death if not urgently treated.

That condition is now quite rare. Its decline may be a result of the widespread use of drugs to control blood pressure, since this acute phase was almost always a complication of long-standing hypertension, which is now being better treated. Some have suggested that the decline cannot be explained entirely by drug therapy. I am reminded about the old experience with rheumatic fever. It is a complication of streptococcus infections and was a common childhood illness before the penicillin era. It has essentially disappeared in advanced societies where antibiotics are readily available. Some think, however, that it began to disappear before antibiotics became available.

Recognition of the urgency of lowering blood pressure in patients with severe or malignant hypertension and manifestations of acute cardiac or vascular damage led to an era in which modest elevations of blood pressure became inappropriately feared. That era is unfortunately not necessarily over. If a patient appears in an emergency room with a systolic blood pressure of greater than 180 mmHg, inexperienced health-care providers may be motivated to give a drug to lower it, even though it is not associated with any signs of distress. They forget that blood pressure levels higher than that are commonplace in our daily lives. During vigorous exercise, the systolic pressure may rise above 200 mmHg because the heart may be pumping five times the resting amount of blood into the arteries. Such readings need not be alarming and certainly need not lead to aggressive treatment. In fact, one of the treatments often used in the past in emergency rooms to acutely lower blood pressure turned out to have more adverse effects than benefits.[9] Except under unusual circumstances, pressure itself is not the problem.

Then why is the level of blood pressure so closely linked to the risk of heart attacks and strokes?

The answer is in the wall of the arteries. Blood pressure is both a marker and a contributor to abnormalities in the artery wall. It is disease of the artery wall that causes heart attacks, strokes, and almost all cardiovascular morbidity. Plaques that obstruct the lumen or channel of the artery, as well as clots that cause heart attacks, always form on an already damaged artery wall. This damage causes thickening and stiffening of the arteries. These changes are what we call arteriosclerosis or atherosclerosis, or the more contemporary term, atherothrombosis. This new term implies that lipid-containing plaques in the artery lead to clots that result in thrombosis (occlusion of the artery) that causes heart attacks and strokes.

These large arteries do not, however, produce resistance to blood flow. If one artery is blocked, there are thousands of parallel channels through which the blood can easily flow. Small arteries, however—the microscopic ones we cannot see—impose a resistance to blood flow that accounts for the head of pressure in the large arteries. If all the body's small artery walls become stiffened or thick, the resistance faced by blood ejected from the heart will be increased and the blood pressure will rise. Small artery disease almost always leads to accelerated large artery disease. Thus elevated blood pressure may be a marker of artery wall disease. The higher the blood pressure, the more likely there is small artery wall disease as well as large artery disease or atherothrombosis.

Elevated blood pressure itself may also over long periods of time further damage the wall of arteries other than the coronary arteries. The higher the pressure, the more likely there will be thickening of the wall, stiffening of the artery, and even rupture of those pesky plaques that lead to clots. So the relationship between blood pressure and morbid events is entirely predictable, both because blood pressure marks the severity of the disease and blood pressure contributes to the severity of the disease.

And remember, the relationship between blood pressure and risk is linear and continuous. There is no threshold for risk. There is no blood pressure level associated with no risk for a heart attack or stroke, only that the risk is somewhat lower when the blood pressure is low and somewhat higher when the blood pressure is high.

This modest relationship between pressure and risk calls into question the guidelines for traditional management of blood pressure. Treatment is recommended when blood pressure is above a certain threshold and not utilized when pressure is below that threshold. Treatment is a binary decision: yes, you treat; no, you don't treat. But the measurement that serves as the guide to treatment is far from binary. The risk is only a little higher or a little lower. And this risk applies to populations, not necessarily to individuals.

A USEFUL ANALOGY?

I always hesitate to use analogies in biology because each biological system is quite unique. But the issue of what is a normal blood pressure and what should be the goal of treatment demands scrutiny.

Let's take as an example the issue of a normal hemoglobin level. Measurement of a patient's hemoglobin is, similar to blood pressure, a standard medical practice technique to assess a patient's health. A low hemoglobin level, below some arbitrary level designed to separate normal from low, establishes the diagnosis of anemia, which usually initiates an evaluation to determine the cause of the anemia and a treatment strategy to correct it.

Biostatisticians can document the fact that in a large population, low hemoglobin levels are predictive of a higher morbidity and mortality rate. Indeed, low hemoglobin is bad for you, not necessarily because of the low hemoglobin itself but, in part, because the low hemoglobin level may be associated with serious diseases that shorten people's lives.

But not everyone with a low hemoglobin level is sick. My wife, for instance, has had a low hemoglobin level for her entire life. It is in the range identified as "anemia." Her sister also has a low hemoglobin level. In the previously mentioned "twin study" carried out at the University of Minnesota, we found a remarkable similarity in hemoglobin values between identical twins raised apart. The body's genome sets the stable level of variables like hemoglobin and blood pressure, which are controlled by physiologic processes that can turn on or turn off the compensatory mechanisms that can influence the levels. My wife doesn't have anemia. Her set point is lower. She doesn't need treatment to reach an arbitrary level of hemoglobin that we have decided is "normal."

In recent years, it was observed that patients with heart failure, who suffer from fatigue presumably because of their heart failure, had lower levels of hemoglobin than individuals without heart failure. Several investigators tried treating these patients to normalize their hemoglobin levels. They claimed in these case reports that the patients exhibited a dramatic improvement in symptoms. Amgen, the pharmaceutical company that manufactures and sells a drug that stimulates the production of hemoglobin, noted that their drug was being prescribed for patients with heart failure even though it was not approved for that condition. Since the potential market for that use could be huge, they decided to fund a study to document the benefits of restoring hemoglobin levels to our arbitrarily determined normal level in patients with heart failure.

This was an ambitious international effort to recruit thousands of patients with heart failure and a low hemoglobin level. Half were randomly assigned to regular injections of darbepoetin, the drug that raises hemoglobin levels, and half to receive placebo injections. Neither the patient nor the caregivers knew which drug the patient received, and the investigators were asked not to measure hemoglobin levels that might have revealed which drug the patient was receiving. Such measurements were made on the patients, but the results were not made available to the doctors or patients. The study went on for years while recruitment and follow-up was completed.

I served as chairman of the Data Monitoring Committee for this study. That means I saw all the data along with my committee members. It was clear from the onset that darbepoetin was producing a dramatic and consistent correction in the low hemoglobin level and the placebo was not. But after years of follow-up, it became apparent that there was no improvement in outcome in response to treatment.[10] Patients neither felt better nor lived longer. Correcting anemia from a low hemoglobin level to what is called a normal level in patients with heart failure was of no therapeutic benefit. Trying to "normalize" abnormal numbers in human disease is not generally a rewarding endeavor.

What about blood pressure? If you are genetically designed to protect a resting blood pressure of 120/80 mmHg, then your blood vessel tone and heart function will be adjusted to that level. Sensors in your arteries are designed to adjust these physiologic variables to maintain that pressure. If, on the other hand, your genes have selected a set point of 140/90 mmHg, there would be no reason to lower the pressure unless there was evidence that the higher pressure was associated with abnormalities of the function or structure of the arteries or heart. It is true that among people with a blood pressure of 140/90 mmHg, a higher proportion will have abnormal arteries than among those with pressures of 120/80 mmHg, but the pressure alone cannot define who has a problem and who does not. Manipulating a number to achieve some arbitrary level of "normalcy" is no more rational for blood pressure than it is for hemoglobin.

The difference between hemoglobin and blood pressure is critical. For hemoglobin, a low level initiates an evaluation. If no abnormal cause, such as blood loss or iron deficiency, is detected, no treatment is offered. For blood pressure, however, an elevated level is treated in order to achieve an arbitrary level considered normal. Despite our sophistication as a medical society, we still rely on a number—which is highly variable and poorly reproducible—to make a diagnosis and treat a patient. Assessment of the health of the arteries and heart would be a far more useful discriminator than the blood pressure itself.

WHAT SHOULD BE THE TARGET FOR THERAPY?

Since the measured blood pressure is usually the sole criterion for initiating therapy to lower it, a level of blood pressure obviously becomes the target for its treatment. Blood pressure is continuously related to risk, so one might assume that management guidelines would set a goal for a low-risk pressure like 120/80 mmHg. But such a goal would conflict with the treatment threshold. How can you advocate for a systolic pressure of 120 mmHg when you do not recommend treatment for 130 or 135 mmHg? The established target for treatment has been to lower the blood pressure below 140/90 mmHg, the same pressure that serves as the threshold for treatment. Obviously, individuals who begin at 142/92 mmHg require less therapy than those who begin at 170/110 mmHg. But the response to drugs is highly variable and the management of hypertension has been largely empirical. There are few clues as to how individuals will respond to specific drugs. Doctors are urged to initiate treatment and observe the response. If the pressure target is not reached, the dose should be increased or another drug should be added.

This treatment strategy once was known as the "stepped care" management of hypertension. Guidelines committees advocated for starting one drug, then adding a second, and then a third or fourth until blood pressure was satisfactorily reduced below the target of 140/90 mmHg and without intolerable side effects. Based on early clinical trial experience, a diuretic, usually hydrochlorthiazide, was recommended as step one and a beta blocker, such as atenolol, as step two. As new antihypertensive drugs became available, tested, and marketed, the guidelines were loosened to allow a variety of drugs to be used as step one, with a diuretic often occupying step two. The goal always was to get pressure below 140/90 mmHg, even if this required high doses of four or more drugs. Because of the power of the guidelines in driving clinical practice, manufacturers of individual drugs put great effort into trying to get their drugs advocated for an early step in the algorithm. More recently the "stepped care" approach has been replaced by a more targeted approach. Starting combination drug therapy is generally encouraged since most patients require more than one drug for optimal control.

The emphasis on target blood pressure satisfied the Food and Drug Administration to allow drug approval based on blood pressure reduction. This was an unusual position for the FDA, since its federal mandate was to approve drugs that improve patient well-being or prognosis. They have vigorously pursued a policy of requiring evidence for patient benefit before drug approval. So in the case of antihypertensive drugs, they had to take the stance that the relationship between blood pressure and morbid events was so persuasive that they were willing to approve drugs that lower blood pressure, with the assumption that they would reduce morbidity, just as the early studies of antihypertensive drugs had succeeded in doing. They had bought into the conventional view that the blood pressure is important and how you reduce it is not.

But as new antihypertensive agents became available, the FDA was becoming growingly uncomfortable with their process. Furthermore, the medical community became more and more focused on preventing heart attacks and strokes, not merely lowering blood pressure. Drug companies realized that sales of their new and expensive drugs would require more than a blood pressure reduction. They had to document that the drugs improved prognosis. But this was difficult to do because patients were already being treated with effective drugs, often now generic and inexpensive. The pharmaceutical industry had to design large studies to document the benefit of their new drugs on outcomes, and they had to design such studies so that everyone was treated with acceptable blood-pressure-lowering therapy. In these trials, the new drugs were generally given in a fixed dose, not titrated to specific blood pressure goals. The question for the sponsor was: if patients take our drug, will they be benefited by fewer morbid events when compared to patients whose blood pressures are similarly controlled without our drug? These studies required thousands of patients and were inordinately expensive. But the billion dollar market for a successful drug made it all worthwhile to the sponsors.

These studies all targeted what drug to take, not what pressure to achieve. The latter question remained unresolved. We had a variety of old and new drugs that were capable of reducing blood pressure, albeit not in a predictable manner. Should we be satisfied with below 140/90 mmHg as the target for therapy or perhaps push for a lower level? After all, blood pressure is continuously related to risk epidemiologically so the thinking was that targeting a lower pressure should further reduce risk. An initial attempt to target a lower blood pressure was carried out in Europe with a trial in which patients were randomly assigned to a group who were treated to a goal of a diastolic pressure of 90 mmHg and a group treated to a goal of 80 mmHg. The latter group obviously required more drugs. Disappointingly, there was no difference in the outcomes between the two groups.[11] But the investigators were not to be deterred. They re-examined their data and discovered that those who achieved a blood pressure of 120/78 mmHg, regardless of which group they were assigned to, had the lowest morbid event rates. They proposed, therefore, that such a blood pressure could serve as a target for therapy.

Such a recommendation fails to appreciate the difference between an association and cause and effect. People whose blood pressure falls in response to simple drug therapy to levels like 120/78 mmHg probably do not have advanced vascular disease. I wonder whether some of them need treatment at all. People who are resistant to drug therapy and require high doses of multiple drugs to achieve adequate blood pressure control probably have advanced disease and are at high risk for heart attacks and strokes. The question is not whether those whose blood pressures fall are at lower risk but whether the effort to further reduce blood pressure will further reduce risk. It did not in this study.

In recent years, several additional trials have been carried out to target lower blood pressures in specific populations. They have all failed and, in some instances, have demonstrated an adverse effect of more aggressive blood pressure control.[12] So the epidemiological data that links blood pressure to outcome in a linear fashion could not be reproduced by lowering blood pressure with the tested drugs. This is hardly surprising, since an artery wall abnormality may cause the rise in blood pressure and some drugs may reduce the blood pressure elevation without correcting the artery wall abnormality.

The uncertainty about the optimal blood pressure target appeared to be resolved in September 2015 with the high-profile report of the 8,000-patient SPRINT Trial, an NIH-sponsored drug intervention trial purported to address whether 140 mmHg or 120 mmHg should be the target for antihypertensive therapy.[13] The investigators were delighted to report that the 120 target saved lives compared to the 140 target. The saving of lives was either related to achieving the lower blood pressure, to giving more drugs to achieve the lower blood pressure, or to both.

I have questioned the selection of patients in the SPRINT study. In order to have enough morbid events to answer the optimal target blood pressure question, they selected individuals at high risk for morbid events, which means that most had already sustained such events. It was therefore largely a secondary prevention study, a population that already had sustained an event and should have been on specific antihypertensive drug therapy regardless of their blood pressure. The study only masqueraded as a blood pressure study. It was actually predominately a study of the prudence of aggressive drug therapy regardless of blood pressure in patients with vascular disease, a strategy that already proved to be effective in several previous long-term trials. The drugs used do indeed lower blood pressure. But their effectiveness in saving lives is that they heal the disease in the arteries and heart that lead to death. Yes, the blood pressure falls, and that's a good sign. But the effectiveness is on the artery wall and heart muscle. The disease in the artery wall often causes the blood pressure to rise. When the rise is to abnormal levels, treatment to lower blood pressure is advocated. But when the rise is less and the blood pressure remains within normal limits, no treatment is recommended. That's a mistake, since the artery wall abnormality in need of treatment exists even though the blood pressure is within normal limits. Most of the patients in SPRINT had advanced artery wall disease, so aggressive treatment with drugs that heal the artery would be expected to be effective. Applying the same strategy to patients with a pressure greater than 120/80 mmHg in the absence of artery wall disease could lead to adverse effects. Guideline committees have yet to grapple with how the SPRINT trial results should influence patient care.

Management strategies based on blood pressure without attention to the presence or absence of artery disease are misguided. In a later chapter, we will explore our approach to identifying that early disease, the disease that makes the patient eligible to join the "club" of those who need treatment to protect their cardiovascular system. Unfortunately for those who make their living treating blood pressure, the pressure itself is an unreliable guide to who needs treatment and therefore an unreliable target for treatment.

Doctors often give patients with high blood pressure the option of taking a drug or drastically altering their lifestyle. Diet and exercise are the two most common recommendations. Salt restriction may lower pressure in some individuals, particularly those who are "salt sensitive"; that is, unable to fully excrete a high salt intake. Weight loss is known to lower blood pressure modestly. Is lowering blood pressure with lifestyle changes equivalent to lowering blood pressure with drugs? That issue has never been addressed in a clinical trial. I don't think they are the same, even if they comparably reduce the pressure. Drugs, especially the newer classes of drugs that are currently in wide use, exert protective effects on the artery above and beyond their blood-pressure-lowering effect. They are not just lowering blood pressure; they are healing the arteries. Whether lifestyle changes can also accomplish that is unknown.

I am convinced that blood pressure is not the disease. It may be a marker for the likelihood of disease and it may contribute to progression of the disease, but using blood pressure as the sole diagnostic criterion for hypertension and as the sole target for therapy is misguided. It fails to recognize most of the population at risk and sets up therapeutic targets that may be ill-advised. Arterial wall disease and atherothrombotic disease are real. They lead to most of the cardiovascular morbidity and mortality in the Western world. They are by far the largest consumers of health-care expenditures in the United States. This vascular disease needs to be aggressively treated. But blood pressure is not an adequate guide to its diagnosis, and blood pressure control is an inadequate guide to its optimal treatment.

HOW TO INTERPRET YOUR OWN BLOOD PRESSURE

Blood pressure is an important and simple measurement that provides insight into the health of your cardiovascular system. But blood pressure is highly variable from moment to moment and must be interpreted in context. You do not have a single blood pressure. It varies throughout the day.

You likely have your blood pressure measured when you visit the doctor. You also may measure it yourself at drug stores and health clubs. You may even buy your own blood pressure device and measure it at home. It is important to recognize that none of these devices is perfect. Most of them these days utilize what is called an oscillometric method. That is, the cuff when placed properly around the upper arm is able to detect movement of the artery that is surrounded by the cuff. When the cuff is inflated to a pressure higher than your blood pressure, the artery is closed by the high pressure. As the cuff gradually deflates, the device detects oscillations in the artery at the point when the cuff pressure falls below the systolic pressure, or the pressure while the heart is contracting. The device identifies this as systolic pressure, the high number in the measurement, because at that point the artery beneath the cuff is opening up when the heart contracts. As the cuff continues deflating, it detects the point where oscillations of the artery no longer occur because the cuff is not occluding the artery even in diastole, just before the next heart contraction. That point is identified as diastolic pressure, or the low number in the measurement.

The problem with all such measurements is that they are indirect. They make the assumption that the pressure in the cuff is transmitted directly to the underlying artery and provides an accurate assessment of pressure exerted on the artery wall. I described earlier in this chapter occasions when this assumption is not true, such as when the arm is fat or severely tapered or the cuff is improperly applied. So with all appropriate caveats that the measurement may not be an accurate estimate of the pressure within the artery, these indirect measurements are all we routinely have available. If your blood pressure is measured by one of these devices as carefully as possible, we must accept that reading as your blood pressure at that moment in time.

The blood pressure varies throughout the day. It is generally at its lowest level during the night and then rises briskly in the morning, often before we arise, and then may gradually fall later in the day. This diurnal variation is not fully understood but probably relates to a predictable pattern of activity of the nervous system and hormone systems. These systems influence the tone or state of constriction of the arteries, and that is probably why the blood pressure varies throughout the day.

If your blood pressure is less than 120/80 mmHg on most of your readings, it is unlikely that you have significant disease in your arteries; not impossible, but unlikely. That doesn't mean you are "home free." Vascular disease develops over time. Even if you have inherited the genetic traits that cause hypertension or vascular disease, your blood pressure may not start rising until your forties or fifties. My own blood pressure was usually about 100/60 mmHg until I was well into my forties, when it began to rise and eventually required treatment. Indeed, both of my parents had hypertension and vascular disease. So whatever blood pressure you have now, it should be tracked, at least annually, to detect changes over time.

If your blood pressure is generally in the range of 120–139/80–89 mmHg, you have what is now often referred to as "pre-hypertension." This is a vague term and an unfortunately misleading one. It is based on the well-established threshold for the diagnosis of hypertension at 140/90 mmHg, so pressures below that range cannot really be called hypertension. But long-term follow-up studies show that people with pressures in that range, as compared to those with optimal pressures below 120/80 mmHg, have a higher risk for heart attacks and strokes. So the experts thought this condition required a name. The term pre-hypertension was probably a poor choice because there was no evidence that the blood pressure actually rose in these individuals before they suffered their morbid events. And no one really suggested that they be treated. That would be heresy since their blood pressure levels were below the ordained threshold for treatment. Unless you are prepared to undergo more extensive testing of the health of your arteries (this will be discussed in a subsequent chapter), pressures in this range should at least alert you to the potential for future problems and encourage you to monitor your pressure more closely.

The reason 135/85 mmHg places you at higher risk than 120/80 mmHg is not necessarily related to the genes that provided you a blood pressure set point. It's really because some people whose set point may have been 120/80 mmHg developed early artery wall abnormalities that caused their blood pressure to rise above their normal set point. Thus the population of people with a blood pressure of 135/85 mmHg contains two subpopulations: one with a genetically determined set point of 135/85 mmHg who are healthy, and one whose normal set point was lower but have now developed early artery disease that is raising their pressure. The only current way to distinguish these groups is by determining the health of the arteries.

If your resting, sitting pressure is generally, or even occasionally, above 140/90 mmHg, medical therapy may be appropriate. This is probably prudent because a majority of such individuals exhibit abnormal artery function or structure, even though some are normal. In the most recent expert guidelines, however, doctors are advised not to initiate therapy in individuals over the age of sixty unless their systolic blood pressure is over 150 mmHg.[14] Unfortunately, not all health-care providers will give you the same advice. Some providers might examine your other risk factors, such as family history, body mass index, and lifestyle, and advise attempts at lifestyle change. Others may merely tell you to come back in six months or a year for re-evaluation. Others may start you on medical treatment. The expert guidelines provide for these options. Can you be sure your doctor is making the right decision? No. Is a more rational decision available? Yes. But you'll have to wait until a later chapter to read about it.

CONTEMPORARY UNDERSTANDING

- Blood pressure levels provide some insight into the health of the arteries—the higher the level the more likely artery disease is present—but it is generally an imprecise guide to an individual's personal likelihood of having disease.
- Very high blood pressures are almost always associated with artery disease and must be treated, but a normal blood pressure does not guarantee good health.
- Antihypertensive drug therapy is aimed at treating the artery, not just lowering blood pressure. Therefore this drug therapy should not be confined to people with levels of blood pressure above an arbitrary threshold.
- Lifestyle adjustments may lower blood pressure, but they may not necessarily improve the health of the arteries.
- Targeting a specific blood pressure goal for treatment may not be the most effective way to administer antihypertensive drugs.

4

CHOLESTEROL

CONVENTIONAL WISDOM

- Elevated cholesterol is an important risk factor for cardiovascular morbid events.
- Cholesterol levels can distinguish individuals at risk for cardiovascular disease from those not at risk.
- Drugs to lower cholesterol should be used exclusively in individuals with an elevated cholesterol level.
- Diet is the best way to deal with high cholesterol, and dietary reduction of cholesterol levels makes the use of drugs unnecessary.
- Since the target for therapy is the reduction in cholesterol, it makes no difference how the reduction is accomplished.

WHY CHOLESTEROL IS IMPORTANT

Cholesterol is a critical component of the plaques that grow inside arteries such as the coronary arteries that nourish the heart, the cerebral arteries that serve the brain, and the femoral arteries that bring blood flow to the legs. These plaques may grow in size and eventually narrow the lumen of the arteries to block the free flow of blood. More often, though, these plaques develop fissures or cracks on their surface that encourage the formation of a superimposed blood clot that acutely obstructs blood flow and causes heart attacks or strokes. In the absence of cholesterol, actually the low-density lipoprotein cholesterol that is often referred to as "bad cholesterol," these plaques cannot form. So cholesterol is obligatory for heart attacks to occur, and in its absence, we would not have most acute cardiovascular morbid events.

But the problem is that cholesterol also is a critical component of the membranes that hold our cells together. In the absence of cholesterol, we could not survive. So the question is not "Can we eliminate bad cholesterol?" but rather "How important is its absolute level?"

The whole idea that cholesterol levels are an important risk factor for atherosclerotic disease was not appreciated until recent years. Probably the most fundamental contribution to our current insights came from the work of Ancel Keys, an epidemiologist and a faculty member at the University of Minnesota before my arrival in 1974. Keys was interested in world populations. He collected data in a number of countries and concluded that average cholesterol levels in these populations were correlated with the risk of cardiovascular morbid events in these populations. By plotting event rates versus mean cholesterol levels, he was able to construct almost a straight-line correlation between the society's average cholesterol level and the event rates.[1] This impressed most of the medical community that high cholesterol levels were dangerous and an important determinant of these morbid events such as heart attacks and strokes. Some old colleagues of Ancel's have in recent years claimed that he intentionally left out data from populations that did not fit onto his straight-line correlation, but even if he doctored the data—and I don't know if he did—the observation probably holds. This and subsequent similar observations in other populations convinced the medical community that elevated cholesterol levels should be lowered.

Dietary indiscretion can raise the blood level of cholesterol. Many foods contain cholesterol itself, which can be absorbed. Saturated fat intake may also raise bad cholesterol levels. The focus on dietary sources of LDL cholesterol has led to widespread recommendations from health authorities to restrict the intake of fats and eggs. The problem is, however, that more cholesterol is manufactured by the body, specifically the liver, than is absorbed from the intestinal tract. Furthermore, when dietary intake of fat is reduced, the body revs up its internal process of synthesis of cholesterol. That partly accounts for why diets low in cholesterol and saturated fats are only modestly if at all effective in lowering the blood level of bad cholesterol. The role of diet in influencing risk will be further considered in a future chapter.

The solution to this problem of lowering cholesterol to reduce risk came in the form of a class of drugs developed by the Nobel Prize–winning team of Michael Brown and Joseph Goldstein. They identified a key enzyme in the liver necessary for production of cholesterol. By inhibiting this enzyme, called HMG Co-A Reductase, they were able to block the synthesis of cholesterol and also to stimulate receptors in the liver that extract bad cholesterol from the blood and turn it into bile.[2] These enzyme inhibitors, called statins, have become the most widely used drugs in the world. Their effectiveness in preventing heart attacks and strokes has focused the medical world's attention on the virtue of reducing elevated levels of cholesterol.

But the story is not as simple as putting Ancel Keys's observation of the adverse consequence of high cholesterol alongside the clinical trial benefits of the statins. The role of cholesterol levels, specifically LDL cholesterol, as a contributor to the frequency of heart attacks is statistically sound and incontrovertible. But the magnitude of the association is quite modest and is continuous from very low levels to very high levels of cholesterol. There is no magical threshold level at which cholesterol becomes dangerous, except perhaps at an LDL cholesterol level of 180 or 190 mg%, which identifies individuals with familial hypercholesterolemia, a condition associated with premature atherosclerosis.[3] And there is certainly no level of cholesterol that is a guarantee of the absence of heart attacks. With strokes, the story is even more confounding. Cholesterol levels are not at all predictive of strokes, but statin drugs are remarkably effective in reducing the risk of strokes. Furthermore, in recent studies carried out specifically in individuals whose cholesterol levels were not elevated, the statin drugs reduced the rates of both heart attacks and strokes.[4] So cholesterol levels are modestly important, but statin drugs work even when the levels are normal and probably exert at least some of their beneficial effect through mechanisms other than cholesterol lowering. Is there an ideal target level for LDL cholesterol that is appropriate for everyone? Probably not.

ARE THE SUBFRACTIONS OF CHOLESTEROL IMPORTANT?

When cholesterol levels in the blood are measured, the components of the cholesterol are identified. Cholesterol doesn't float in blood by itself but is linked to a protein that holds it in a particle within the blood stream. Some of the cholesterol in the blood is transported in particles with a low density of protein, the low density lipoprotein (LDL). These particles easily give up their cholesterol to invade the artery wall. Thus the term "bad cholesterol" is used. Some of the cholesterol is transported in particles with high density lipoprotein, HDL, which is often identified as "good cholesterol." These particles do not release their cholesterol into the artery wall, and in fact tend to take up some of the excess LDL in the arteries to transport it to the liver for excretion in the bile.

Triglycerides are another form in which fat is transported in the blood. Since about 20 percent of the triglycerides are made up of cholesterol, it is customary when assessing an individual's cholesterol level to assume that one-fifth of the triglyceride concentration consists of cholesterol that is neither "bad" LDL cholesterol nor "good" HDL cholesterol. In fact, we still are uncertain if the cholesterol in triglycerides does any harm to the blood vessels. We do know, however, that high triglyceride levels are associated with more cardiovascular disease. One explanation for that is that high triglycerides are often associated with low "good" HDL levels, so the adverse effects may be related to the low HDL rather than to the triglycerides themselves.

When laboratories analyze blood for cholesterol levels, they usually measure the total cholesterol (which is LDL + HDL), they measure the HDL, and they measure the triglycerides. The LDL is calculated, not measured, as the total cholesterol minus the HDL minus 20 percent of the triglycerides. From a statistical standpoint, your chances of having atherosclerosis that can lead to a heart attack or stroke is lower if your LDL is low, your HDL is high, and your triglycerides are not elevated. High levels of LDL increase your risk, low levels of HDL increase your risk, and high levels of triglycerides may increase your risk, but these risk increases are quite small. They certainly do not tell you if you do or do not have atherosclerotic disease. Like the barometer in predicting a storm, it is less likely to rain if the barometric pressure is high, but if a black cloud is overhead, you should carry an umbrella.

In recent years, this simple concept that the ratio of LDL to HDL is an important predictor of atherosclerosis has been challenged. Drugs that raise HDL levels, and there have been several, have failed to improve outcomes. It is now recognized that all HDL is not protective. Many individuals and families have very high levels of HDL that are not protective, so the idea that a high HDL keeps you safe is no longer tenable. Since the laboratory testing of cholesterol provides several numbers that can be manipulated, the current fashion is to subtract HDL from total cholesterol and report a number called "non-HDL cholesterol." Some think that is a more accurate way to calculate the adverse effect of cholesterol on risk. It has really become a numbers game.

Lipoprotein(a) or LP(a) is a subfraction of cholesterol that is not routinely measured in blood samples but can be analyzed by special laboratories. It appears to be especially predictive of atherosclerotic disease. High levels greater than 50 mg% are better correlated with atherosclerosis than are high levels of the routinely measured LDL. Not much is known about how to modify LP(a) levels or how it directly influences plaque formation, but it does serve as a statistically significant risk factor. Should it be measured routinely? Like all such risk factors, it provides at best statistical likelihood. It's not the disease. That is in the artery wall and can be detected. Detection is a better strategy than risk assessment.

Do doctors put too much faith in the predictive value of cholesterol levels? Do they inappropriately reassure patients whose levels are in the normal range and generate unnecessary anxiety in those with elevated levels? Probably so, but they have been brainwashed by the establishment.

DRUGS THAT LOWER CHOLESTEROL LEVELS

The remarkable success of statin drugs to both lower bad cholesterol and prevent heart attacks and strokes has made this class of drugs one of the most widely used and, at least before they became generic, most lucrative in the pharmaceutical industry. Because statins, like all drugs, may produce unwanted side effects in some individuals and because statins do not relieve symptoms or improve quality of life, their widespread use has resulted in many reports of adverse effects. Some of these adverse effects are drug-related, but many may be the consequence of individual's attributing a minor symptom to a drug of which they were already suspicious. In controlled trials, where patients do not know whether they are receiving active drug or placebo, the rate of side effects in the statin-treated groups is only slightly higher than in the placebo groups. Nonetheless, we know that in some patients an acute and severe inflammatory process in the skeletal muscles may be precipitated by statins, and in others muscle aches of a more mild form may be associated with taking the drug. In those instances, it is usually appropriate to discontinue the statin drug, or at least to very cautiously switch to a different member of the class.

Fortunately, the pharmaceutical industry's creativity is most evident when they have an established target for drug therapy. Statins target the synthesis of cholesterol, which involves a complex series of chemical steps. Ezetimibe, or Zetia, targets not the synthesis of cholesterol but its absorption from food in the gut. Two new injectable drugs—alirocumab, or Praluent, and evolucamab, or Repatha—target a different step in synthesis and produce a profound reduction in the blood levels of bad cholesterol. They have just been approved by the FDA even without the demonstration of cardiovascular morbid event prevention that many experts think should have been required.

Supporters of the cholesterol hypothesis would insist that lowering bad cholesterol levels will always reduce the risk of heart attacks and strokes. They would like to think that high cholesterol is the disease. They often suggest to patients that they should try diet to lower their cholesterol rather than take a drug, with the assumption that how you lower cholesterol is less important than that the level falls. They would like to think that any familial incidence of heart attacks and strokes is due to inheritance of an elevated cholesterol level. If that were true, of course, then all patients with heart attacks would have a high cholesterol level and all treatments that lower cholesterol would have a similar effect on preventing these heart attacks.

The facts don't support this argument. The vast majority of patients who have heart attacks have bad cholesterol levels within the so-called normal range. That argument is discounted by the advocates with the claim, supported in guidelines, that the target level of bad cholesterol should be well below the "normal range." A more persuasive argument comes from the evidence that different cholesterol-lowering therapy exhibits differential benefit on heart attacks and strokes. Statins produce a dramatic benefit on outcomes, even when administered to patients with normal levels of bad cholesterol. In contrast, Zetia appears to have at best a very slight effect on morbid events, even though bad cholesterol levels are markedly decreased.[5] The new drugs, Praluent and Repatha, have a profound lowering effect on LDL cholesterol but have not yet been subjected to an adequate long-term trial to evaluate for morbid events.

So there is nothing wrong with dietary efforts to lower cholesterol, although they are rarely successful. But to be assured that an intervention is slowing progression of atherosclerosis, statins should be employed if they are tolerated.

OTHER FACTORS CAUSING MORBID EVENTS

While a cholesterol-containing atherosclerotic plaque on the inner lining of an artery is a prerequisite for most heart attacks and strokes, the presence of such plaques does not necessarily result in these morbid events. Autopsies performed in centenarians who have never suffered from cardiovascular morbid events often reveal extensive atherosclerotic plaques in the aorta and coronary arteries. What else is needed in addition to the plaques?

Most morbid events result from rupture or fracture of these atherosclerotic plaques. This rupture exposes the flowing blood to chemicals that encourage the platelets in the blood to aggregate or congeal, thus initiating the process of clot formation that usually causes the morbid event. This process may be a consequence of inflammation in the plaque itself, perhaps enhanced when the plaque contains lots of cholesterol or lipid and has not hardened over with calcium. So drugs that interfere with this inflammatory process or discourage platelet aggregation may prevent heart attacks, even if the plaque is already there. Therefore, heart attacks occur only if there are plaques in a coronary artery, but all plaques do not cause heart attacks.

Data on the effects of statins support the idea that some of their benefit is not just a result of a reduction in bad cholesterol levels but also related to what are called "pleotropic effects," that is, a second effect independent of their action to reduce bad cholesterol levels. It is this pleotropic effect, which is probably missing from Zetia, that accounts for why its effect on morbid events is so feeble compared to the statins. It raises concerns about new drugs that are effective in lowering cholesterol. And it obviously raises the important issue of whether dietary reduction of bad cholesterol, if it can be accomplished, would have a benefit on outcome anywhere near as great as that from the statins.

WHO SHOULD BE TREATED WITH STATINS?

The remarkable benefit of statin drugs, even when cholesterol levels are normal, should mandate that all individuals with early disease, such as plaques, likely to progress should be treated with a statin drug. Such therapy is now mandated in guidelines for individuals who have had a heart attack or stroke, obviously evidence for atherosclerotic disease.

Is it appropriate to use blood cholesterol levels to determine who should be given a statin drug? Is an elevated LDL cholesterol enough to make you a member of the "club" that needs treatment? The answer is probably "yes" if the level is very high, above 190 mg%. Individuals with such high LDL levels probably have an inherited, familial form of hyper-lipidemia that is associated with a high risk for future cardiovascular morbid events. These individuals may be accepted into the "club" without any additional testing, although some of them may still be remarkably free from apparent artery wall abnormalities. Their statistical risk is high enough to justify treatment.

Guidelines are now unclear about what to do with elevated LDL levels that do not reach this high threshold. They recommend assessing risk based on risk algorithms constructed from large databases of historical data, which usually includes age, gender, blood pressure, and cholesterol levels. If the risk by this statistical analysis is high—somewhere between 7.5 and 15 percent over the ensuing ten years—the guidelines recommend consideration of drugs to lower cholesterol if the LDL is greater than 130 mg%. They also encourage target levels of bad cholesterol as the thera-peutic goal, even though the cholesterol level itself does not define who should be treated. The field has become confused by data that contradicts the prior "wisdom" that cholesterol elevation was the disease and the goal of treatment was to lower the cholesterol.

Are higher doses of statins more effective than lower doses? They appear to be, but the data are not entirely clear. Does the higher dose produce greater pleotropic effects, or is the higher dose working through LDL-cholesterol reduction? Studies with the new and more potent LDL-cholesterol-reducing drugs may ultimately demonstrate whether it is cholesterol we should target specifically or whether it is multiple effects that cannot be achieved by reducing cholesterol alone.

Our current approach is to identify early disease in the arteries and heart, regardless of the cholesterol levels. Patients with early disease are in need of statin therapy. They have joined the "club" who need treatment, and statins are one of the treatments aimed at members of the "club." This approach will be discussed in more depth in a subsequent chapter.

CONTEMPORARY UNDERSTANDING

- Elevated bad cholesterol and reduced good cholesterol are modest risk factors for the occurrence of cardiovascular morbid events.
- Other factors, including genetic factors not manifested in cholesterol levels, probably play a more important role and account for why most heart attacks and strokes occur in individuals whose cholesterol levels are not elevated.
- Statin drugs lower cholesterol levels and also greatly reduce the risk of heart attacks and strokes.
- The focus for management should be to identify individuals with early disease (plaques or their precursors) and treat those at-risk individuals with statins, regardless of their level of cholesterol.

5

BLOOD CLOTS

CONVENTIONAL WISDOM

- Blood clots obstruct the flow of blood in arteries and veins.
- Clots in the coronary artery cause heart attacks.
- Clots in the cerebral arteries cause strokes.
- Drugs are effective in dissolving clots and in preventing clots.
- All adults should take low-dose aspirin to prevent clots from forming.

THE REMARKABLE BLOOD-CLOTTING SYSTEM

It is a remarkable tribute to animal design that blood stays fluid inside the blood vessel walls but clots when it escapes. We wouldn't live very long if that miraculous magic of nature did not exist. Yet sometimes the system goes awry. Blood vessels hemorrhage when we don't want them to, and blood clots form when we wish they hadn't.

These errors of health maintenance are explainable. If a blood vessel ruptures, blood leaks out and damages surrounding tissue until the clotting mechanisms are activated to shut off the leakage from the artery wall. And clots sometimes form inside the artery, where we expect blood to flow freely, because of the release of substances that encourage clotting, substances that aren't supposed to be there. These substances include components of cholesterol plaques that get exposed when the surface of the plaque cracks or ruptures. These clots are the cause of a majority of heart attacks and strokes, and our goal should be to prevent them without putting patients at an unacceptably increased risk for hemorrhage.

Acute treatment of the unwanted clot has become a standard treatment strategy in contemporary management of heart attacks and strokes. Time is of the essence, and most major medical centers have developed emergency teams that can render acute care to dissolve the unwanted clots or to open the offending artery with a balloon and stent. The sooner the task is accomplished, the less damage the clot does and the better the prognosis of the patient for recovery. Such management is well reimbursed by health insurance.

There are risks and benefits to all efforts at eliminating clots that obstruct arteries. Drugs like tPA (tissue plasminogen activator) and streptokinase can be administered intravenously or directly into the obstructed artery. They activate an enzyme, plasmin, that breaks down the clot and can restore blood flow. In comparative trials, it has become clear that emergency intervention with a balloon to squash the clot and a stent to keep the artery open is more effective than these drugs at promptly restoring blood flow and relieving symptoms. But how any health-care institution handles such emergencies is very dependent on the facilities and expertise available locally at the time of the event.

Preventing these clots from forming is a more attractive strategy, but the medical establishment has not placed as great an emphasis on this effort, perhaps because there is no reimbursement for preventing clots from forming. I am not suggesting that the health-care system is mercenary, but all systems are built around incentives for good work and rewards for success. There is no reward system for prevention in the current health-care system.

Since the potentially lethal clots form in arteries supplying the heart or brain, the drugs that are useful in preventing these occlusions are inhibitors of platelet activity and do not include the old standby anticoagulants, such as warfarin or Coumadin. Those drugs work by inhibiting thrombin, a constituent of clots, and their action is particularly effective when blood clots in a vascular structure with low or stagnant flow. That's why these drugs are used to prevent clotting in leg veins and in the upper chamber of the heart, or atrium, when the chamber is quivering rather than actively pumping blood because of atrial fibrillation.

Clots in the coronary and cerebral arteries occur because platelets, the tiny particles that circulate in the blood, aggregate or clump. As noted above, this may be due to interaction with substances from cholesterol plaques that grow inappropriately in the artery wall. Preventing this process requires inhibiting platelet aggregation, which warfarin and all the new heavily advertised anticoagulants designed to replace warfarin do not do. That opens the door for aspirin.

WHAT ABOUT ASPIRIN?

Aspirin prevents clots from forming on the wall of the arteries at the site of cholesterol plaques. It produces that effect in low doses, so even a baby aspirin is effective in inhibiting platelet aggregation. Many adults take a baby aspirin daily, either at the advice of their doctor or because of widespread lay media recommendations that it will prevent heart attacks.

Considerable controversy about the prudence of aspirin therapy to prevent heart attacks has developed over recent years.[1] Most often the controversy has revolved around benefit/risk analysis. Aspirin prevents clots from forming at the site of plaques, but it also inhibits clotting elsewhere, such as at the site of injuries, in the brain, and in the intestinal wall. Even a baby aspirin a day produces a surprisingly high incidence of life-threatening or cosmetically unpleasant bleeding and bruising. Is the benefit on preventing heart attacks worth accepting the risk of unwanted bleeding?

Traditional thought was that in individuals who have already suffered a heart attack and were therefore at heightened risk for a subsequent event, aspirin was certainly worth the bleeding risk. For so-called primary prevention, in individuals without a prior history of cardiovascular disease, there was less certainty. But all the large-scale studies of aspirin in the prevention of cardiovascular morbid events were conducted before the current era of statin therapy. Do statin drugs so reduce the likelihood of unstable or fissured plaques that the risk of a heart attack is now lower than the risk of taking aspirin?

The answer to this dilemma is not yet available. It would be very difficult to mount a contemporary study to address this issue, but until such a study is conducted, the use of aspirin will remain an individual doctor and individual patient's prerogative. What do I recommend to my patients? For those who are at risk for a heart attack but are taking chronic statin therapy, I generally do not advise prophylactic aspirin use. That's because I believe that long-term use of statins so reduces the risk of plaque rupture that I think the risk of aspirin overwhelms the benefit.

It is important to point out the contrasting strategies of use of aspirin and statin for prevention of heart attacks. Aspirin targets the clot. It has no effect on the atherosclerotic process. Its sole action is to prevent a heart attack. Every day that passes without a heart attack is a day you didn't need and couldn't have benefited from aspirin. The useless advice: only take aspirin the day you would otherwise have a heart attack. Taking an aspirin at the first sign of a heart attack is good advice, but it always would have been better to prevent it in the first place.

In contrast, statins prevent the build-up of cholesterol plaques that may eventually rupture or obstruct blood flow. Every day you don't take a statin is a day that your plaques, if they exist, may be growing. If you are a member of the "club" who has artery disease, you should take a statin.

A host of new drugs that inhibit platelet activity have entered clinical practice in recent years.[2] They are more potent than aspirin and are often prescribed in high-risk situations, such as when a stent has been placed in the coronary and may be at risk for clotting. Clopidogrel was the first of these drugs, and it is still in wide use. These drugs are linked to a higher incidence of unwanted bleeding than is aspirin, so their use is confined to individuals in whom clotting is a far higher risk than bleeding.

WHAT ABOUT EMBOLIC EVENTS?

Clots not only form in arteries, veins, or the heart chambers, but they may also be propelled with blood flow to distant organs. These embolic events account for many strokes and probably a few heart attacks. They are the major cause of pulmonary embolism, that condition resulting from clots usually formed in leg veins that travel with blood flow back to the right ventricle from which they are ejected into the arteries to the lung. This is a potentially lethal illness that requires all the savvy of emergency medical care.

Normal heart valves are not the site of clot formation that can embolize, but prosthetic heart valves implanted to replace a diseased valve can be the site of clot formation. That is why warfarin is mandated long-term therapy in patients with prosthetic valves. Since the newer anticoagulant drugs have not yet been tested in such patients, the advertising for these drugs as an embolic event preventer in people with atrial fibrillation is obligated to state that the drugs should not be used when atrial fibrillation is caused by valvular disease or in the presence of a prosthetic valve implanted to replace a damaged one.

STROKES AND TIAs

Most strokes are caused by clots in the cerebral arteries. TIAs, or transient ischemic attacks, are thought to be the consequence of small fragments of a clot breaking off from where it has formed on a plaque in a cerebral artery and embolizing or flowing with the bloodstream to lodge in a small branch of the artery where it obstructs blood flow to a tiny region of the brain. The treatment of choice for such TIAs is, of course, aspirin.

The downside of this management is hemorrhage. Although clots in the cerebral arteries are destructive, hemorrhage in the brain is usually worse. So the dilemma is always to weigh the benefits of aspirin, or any other anticoagulant, with the risk of hemorrhage. In the coronary circulation, there is little risk of hemorrhage, but in the cerebral circulation, it is a constant concern.

There is no question that clots kill more people than bleeding does, but the goal of modern medicine is to individualize. Personalized or precision medicine mandates that decisions about use of preventive therapy should be based not only on historical statistical data but on an understanding of an individual's unique risk. For example, I am loath to prescribe an anticoagulant or even aspirin for an avid motorcyclist or an aggressive skier who is prone to accidents. I am sensitive to the vanity of individuals who complain bitterly about unsightly bruising from daily use of aspirin. All of these considerations should be kept in mind in making decisions when the benefit of a therapy is counterbalanced by a risk that is almost as big—and sometimes bigger.

CONTEMPORARY UNDERSTANDING

- Clots in arteries result from platelet aggregation whereas clots in veins and the heart are more dependent on thrombin.
- Drugs can alter the balance between clotting and bleeding.
- The decision to use such drugs requires insight into an individual's unique disease process as well as their personal risk and tolerance to unwanted hemorrhagic events.

6

OBESITY

CONVENTIONAL WISDOM

- Excess body weight is a major cause of cardiovascular disease.
- Obesity can be eliminated by dietary restriction and exercise.
- Obesity is a self-inflicted disease whose control could greatly reduce the epidemic of cardiovascular disease in American society.
- Excess fat consumption is a major contributor to obesity.
- Fat people have higher cholesterol levels than thin people.
- Fat people die younger than thin people.
- Reducing weight in an obese individual will reduce their risk of cardio-vascular disease.

THE SOCIAL STIGMA OF OBESITY

Many years ago I hired a morbidly obese person. I was recruiting for an individual with administrative and accounting skills to oversee the budget of my cardiovascular program. Of all the applicants, the one with the best education and experience was very obese. She weighed well over 300 pounds, and most of it appeared to be fat. But she was very well-spoken and apparently very knowledgeable and competent. I sensed that this job was perhaps below her skill level but that her personal appearance may have forced her to seek a lower-profile position. I offered her the job.

I of course never discussed her obesity with her, since the subject was taboo in the employer-employee relationship, but I silently worried about the appearance of this overweight individual as the public face of a cardiology program. She apparently was sensitive to this unspoken concern and on her own arranged the cabinetry in her office so that she was hidden from the hallway. She was probably well aware of the social stigma of her obesity.

Unfortunately her performance did not match her potential. After a few months, it became apparent that her skill set was not a good fit with her responsibilities. We mutually agreed on her termination, not because she was obese but because she was not capable. I never saw or heard from her again. I don't know if she found another position, but I knew that wherever she worked she would face the same obesity issue in the workplace.

This experience informed me about the social stigma obese people face. It convinced me, if I had needed convincing, that obesity should be vigorously avoided, not only for potential health issues but for its potentially adverse effect on quality of life.

IS OBESITY A RISK FACTOR FOR DISEASE?

All the stories about the health dangers of obesity are not wrong. Over-abundant weight gain, whether behavioral or genetic, carries with it a greater risk for a number of medical problems, certainly including cardiovascular diseases. Obesity burdens the heart by an excess demand for tissue nourishment, especially with weight-bearing activity. But obese individuals who develop heart failure, perhaps a consequence in part of that excess demand, actually live longer than thin people who develop heart failure. That surprising but reproducible observation has been called "the obesity paradox," and it remains not fully explained. I view it as likely due to the fact that obesity precipitates heart failure at an earlier stage of the heart disease. The observation should not, however, be used to encourage people to gain weight. Association does not imply cause and effect.

The mechanism by which obesity leads to excess disease in the arteries is not clear. There is no question that obese individuals have a statistically higher risk of developing heart attacks and strokes than that of similarly aged thin individuals. But the magnitude of this increase is really quite modest. Don't get me wrong. From the population standpoint a 5 or 10 percent increase in morbid event rates can have a profound effect on the cost of health care. Since cardiovascular health-care costs exceed $1 trillion a year, 10 percent of that could account for a $100 billion increase in cost attributed to cardiovascular care in the American population. But when it comes to an individual, a 10 percent increase in risk is barely discernible. It might raise an individual's risk from 1 in 10 to 1 in 9, hardly a change likely to be noticed. Furthermore, we don't know if it's the obesity itself or the genetics of the individual who tends to get obese. We don't know if weight loss in an obese patient reduces his or her risk. Attempts to document that in well-controlled trials have usually failed. The risk may not be the obesity itself, but the metabolic derangement that makes obesity likely. Individuals destined to be obese may exhibit the same risk if they become obese or if they stay trim.

The best attempt to answer this unresolved question was published in 2016.[1] A group of Swedish investigators took advantage of the remarkable national database available in Sweden to examine outcomes in identical twins. They focused on thousands of identical twins whose body weight or body mass index differed widely. If weight differs in identical twins, the difference must be environmental because they both have the exact same genome. By focusing on the obese and thin pairs, they studied the medical illnesses and deaths experienced during their lives. The obese individuals developed more diabetes, a condition we will explore in the next chapter and one identified by a high blood sugar that is critically dependent on diet. But there was no excess of cardiovascular events in the obese twins compared to their thin siblings. This study would appear to confirm the opinion that dietary indiscretion may not accelerate cardiovascular disease. The genetic background that encourages obesity may accelerate the disease, but it may not be the diet or the obesity itself.

So the answer is that obesity is clearly a population risk, but it's at most only a small factor in determining individual risk. And we're not sure if it is the obesity itself. The blame placed on lifestyle-induced obesity for the frequency of heart disease in America may be overemphasized.

WHY DOES OBESITY INCREASE RISK?

The best explanation for the adverse effects of obesity on cardiovascular health relates to the endothelium, that single layer of cells that line the inside of all arteries. Knowledge about the endothelium has exploded in the past twenty years, thanks to innovative studies by a number of vascular scientists.[2] Endothelial cells are highly specialized structures that serve as a barrier between the blood circulating in the arteries and the underlying arterial wall. The barrier function of these cells is dependent on a substance, actually a gas, released from the endothelial cells. This gas protects the artery wall from penetration of particles in the blood, such as cholesterol attached to protein, and also inhibits clotting factors, such as platelets, from blocking the lumen of these arteries and thus interrupting blood flow. Through the efforts of a number of laboratories, this substance was identified as nitric oxide.

We now know that the ability of the endothelial cell to release nitric oxide is a critical determinant of cardiovascular health. It also is a critical factor in male erectile function. With age, there appears to be a gradual decline in this ability, probably a factor in why cardiovascular disease and erectile dysfunction increase progressively with age. Some individuals exhibit a premature decline in endothelial function and may develop impotence. Heredity certainly plays a role in endothelial dysfunction, and the search for a genomic profile of nitric oxide deficiency or endothelial dysfunction goes on. But environmental factors also play a role. Smoking clearly impairs endothelial function.[3] A high-fat diet may also do it.[4] And obese individuals, whether because of a genetic predilection or because of their lifestyle or their obesity itself, also may more commonly exhibit nitric oxide deficiency. This endothelial dysfunction places them at a higher risk for cardiovascular disease. So if it was possible to restore nitric oxide function in obese individuals, one might be able to reduce their risk even though they remained obese. There may be more than one way to solve the problem.

Obesity and cholesterol levels are not really linked. Obesity is often accompanied by an elevated triglyceride level, not an elevated LDL cholesterol, or bad cholesterol, level. Obese individual's HDL cholesterol, or good cholesterol, may be reduced. When an individual has an increased waist circumference accompanied by elevated triglycerides or reduced HDL, and often accompanied by mildly elevated blood pressure and blood sugar levels, they may be diagnosed with "metabolic syndrome," a condition associated with increased risk for cardiovascular disease. Is that increased risk mediated by their cholesterol abnormalities, their obesity, their lifestyle, their ancestors, or all of these, or something else? Journals and societies have sprung up to focus on metabolic syndrome.

We don't know whether nitric oxide deficiency accounts for most of the risk increase, and we don't know the best way to reduce that risk. Experts will advise such individuals to aggressively diet and exercise. That might reduce the risk in a population of individuals with metabolic syndrome. It might improve the quality of life as well. For some individuals, however, it might induce anxiety because of their inability to follow the advice and their growing concern about individual risk, which may in some be unaffected by their "metabolic syndrome." Rather than treating obese individuals on the basis of population data, our approach has been to determine whether these individuals do or do not have early disease. Once again, we should be treating the individual, not the population. This approach will be discussed in detail in a later chapter.

WHAT IS OBESITY?

How do we define obesity? It's like the old story of pornography: "I know it when I see it."

But we need objective criteria by which to define a continuum of weight or body shape that justifies the designation "obese."

Body mass index, or BMI, is the standard criterion. It is a calculation based on height and weight that computes the weight (usually in kilograms) per height (usually in meters). A value higher than 30 is generally defined as "obese." But it is obvious that any arbitrary threshold for an abnormality is just that, arbitrary. Some people with BMI of 31 appear fat, but others do not. It is dependent on the distribution of their fat and muscle mass. In order to assess body shape, there is growing interest in using waist circumference, since abdominal obesity, the classical "apple" shape instead of the "pear" shape, appears to be the culprit. A waist circumference greater than 40 inches in men and greater than 35 inches in women is generally classified as "obese."

There is nothing magical about these arbitrary criteria. A so-called disease, obesity, does not go away if BMI falls from 31 to 29 or if waist circumference decreases from 41 to 39. The arbitrary thresholds serve to assess population statistics and allow us to analyze groups of people with similar body sizes. Once again, however, just like the thresholds for blood pressure and cholesterol, they mean far less for individual health than the population statistics suggest.

WHAT CAUSES OBESITY?

It is a truism that weight gain comes from consuming more calories than one uses up. So every rational book about obesity advises individuals to eat less, exercise more, or do both.

How important is what you eat? Other than quantity, probably not very much. In general, obese individuals consume more carbohydrate, not necessarily more fatty foods. The common pictures of obese individuals in low-income neighborhoods emphasize that caloric intake is not necessarily expensive. Carbohydrates are a cheap source of calories, and the body's craving for salt and sugar can easily be met by carbohydrates rich in seasoning. These processed foods are of course the bane of nutritionists' efforts to curb obesity.

The media and public health agencies have promoted the idea that obesity is the major cause of our epidemic of cardiovascular disease and appear to subtly suggest that if we could eliminate obesity, everyone would live to a ripe old age. These efforts at oversimplification to gain adherence may be an appropriate strategy to get patients involved in the one thing they can do. But the message is unfortunately misleading. It is true that our lifestyle and dietary habits encourage more obesity in the Western world. It is true that this epidemic of obesity may somewhat increase the incidence of cardiovascular disease morbid events. But atherosclerosis, the disease that accounts for most morbid events, is not a modern disease. Recent imaging studies of forty- and fifty-year-old Egyptian mummies have revealed evidence of extensive coronary vascular disease.[5] Even more dramatic was the discovery of extensive atherosclerosis in the body of a 5,300-year-old Tyrolean iceman mummy.[6] Who says atherosclerosis is a complication of dietary indiscretion in our modern era of processed foods and inactivity?

The rarity of heart attacks and strokes in those eras, if indeed they were actually so rare, is probably related to that population's markedly shorter life span. We now live decades longer than the Egyptians did in their era. Our efforts to expand cardiovascular health through the tenth decade of life will require a lot more than controlling obesity. It will require an understanding of the processes that accelerate cardiovascular disease and a recognition of those in whom the process is beginning to progress. It is early recognition and individualized intervention. It is determining who has joined the "club." It is no longer a population problem; it is an individual problem.

OBESITY AND WORKLOAD

Most of our daily activity and exercise is carried out during weight bearing in the upright position. Therefore, body weight is a critical determinant of workload. A 200-pound individual walking up a flight of stairs is doing twice as much work as a 100-pounder. That excess work requires more oxygen delivered to the exercising muscles, which means more blood pumped by the heart. That extra heart work may account in part for why obese individuals are more likely to develop heart failure, and why—if heart failure occurs with lesser underlying heart disease—obese individuals with heart failure live longer than thin individuals with heart failure.

The extra heart work of obese individuals may have other consequences. Exercise tests are often utilized by physicians to assess the health of the heart. The standard exercise test on a treadmill burdens the obese individual far more than a thin individual. This difference in workload is seldom considered in the evaluation of test results. Does it account for the perception that obesity is commonly associated with heart disease? Probably not, but it may play a contributory role.

IS OBESITY INHERITED OR ENVIRONMENTAL?

The emphasis in the media and from health agencies is that obesity is a manifestation of poor personal decisions on diet and activity, but the familial prevalence of obesity is hard to deny. We are all familiar with the sight of obese parents and obese children gathered together at parks and restaurants. Is obesity a condition largely inherited through the genome?

We know that obesity results from consuming more calories than are burned in daily living, but the body establishes set points that seem to balance hunger and satiety. Those set points may be determined by the genes even if they are under the influence of psychological factors and messages sent to the brain from other cells in the body, even fat cells themselves. Some genetic disturbances are known to result in morbid skinniness, and some undoubtedly underlie morbid obesity. Our limitation in understanding the biological pathways that control that genetically determined set point probably accounts for why efforts to reverse obesity have been so unsuccessful.

This is where our understanding of the biological progression of cardiovascular disease gives us an advantage. Even if we do not understand what underlies the atherosclerotic process to set it in motion any more than obesity experts understand what determines the weight set point, we do understand many of the mechanisms of the progression of the process. We also have drugs that can effectively slow that process. We are therefore better able to prevent cardiovascular disease than obesity.

REVERSAL OF OBESITY

Dieting can have a profound effect on weight. When associated with increased exercise, massively obese individuals can be restored to normal weight. Commercial enterprises dedicated to selling their methodology regale us with stories and pictures of their successes. Does such weight loss reverse the adverse effects of obesity on cardiovascular health?

It is hard to know. Blood pressure may come down, triglyceride levels may fall, and diabetes (see below) may disappear, so this reduction in risk factors may lead to claims that cardiovascular disease will be lessened. But documentation of this effect is harder to come by. Obese individuals may be genetically different than thin individuals, and this genetic difference will not be altered by weight loss. A definitive clinical trial comparing long-term outcome of individuals randomly assigned to weight loss vs. not assigned to weight loss would be required. Such a study—which is unlikely to be feasible and unlikely to be designed and carried out— would require thousands of participants. Until that time, the answer to the effectiveness of weight loss on long-term outcome will remain uncertain.

The most robust effort so far was carried out over nearly ten years in more than five thousand patients with diabetes accompanied by obesity. The results of this trial, Look AHEAD, which was funded by the National Institutes of Health, was reported in 2013 in the *New England Journal of Medicine*.[7] By focusing on diabetics with obesity, they assumed they would be intervening on a particularly high-risk population. They randomly assigned these individuals to one of two groups: an aggressive intervention group treated with diet and exercise conditioning and a non-aggressive group given only educational material. The intervention group lost weight and their cardiovascular risk factors were improved, but there was absolutely no difference in the frequency of heart attacks and strokes over the nearly ten years of follow-up.

Should we therefore assume that these costly and time-consuming efforts to lose weight do no good? Perhaps a longer follow-up is necessary to bring out the benefits. Or perhaps the underlying diabetes in these individuals reduced the benefit of weight loss. Perhaps the recent enthusiasm for bariatric surgery will lead to careful follow-up to document if the risk of cardiovascular events has been reduced by the resultant weight loss. Or perhaps waiting for a heart attack or stroke is a too-insensitive test of the benefit. A more attractive strategy might be to evaluate the effect of weight loss on the severity of early cardiovascular disease. That approach would be feasible and could be conducted effectively on a much smaller sample size. If weight loss improved the health of the arteries and heart, we could appropriately speculate that it would reduce the frequency of cardiovascular morbid events.

But based on current evidence, the best we can say with confidence about obesity is that weight loss improves self-respect and quality of life. We cannot defend with scientific evidence the claim implicit in much of the marketing effort from public health agencies that weight loss will improve an individual's cardiovascular health.

CONTEMPORARY UNDERSTANDING

- Obese individuals are on average at higher risk than thin individuals for cardiovascular disease, but it is not known if it is the obesity itself or some other trait associated with the obesity.

- Diet can reverse the obesity, but it is uncertain if weight loss restores the individual to a lower risk.
- Obesity is at least in part self-inflicted, but it is not proved whether it is the lifestyle alone that is responsible.
- Most obesity can be traced to excess carbohydrate, not increased fat, in the diet.
- Bad cholesterol levels (LDL) in the blood are not related to obesity, but triglycerides often are.
- Although obese individuals may die on average at a younger age than thin individuals, there is no evidence that reducing weight prolongs life.

7

DIABETES

CONVENTIONAL WISDOM

- Diabetes is defined by an abnormally elevated blood sugar level.
- An unhealthy lifestyle is an important contributor to the growing risk of diabetes in America.
- The presence of diabetes establishes an individual as at high risk for cardiovascular disease, including heart attacks, strokes, peripheral vascular disease, and kidney disease.
- The risk of a first heart attack in a diabetic is the same as the risk for a second heart attack in a nondiabetic individual who has already had one.
- Controlling blood sugar with drugs or lifestyle reduces the risk of heart attacks, strokes, and kidney disease.
- Weight control and exercise are critical in reducing the cardiovascular risk in diabetics.

WHAT IS DIABETES?

Diabetes is a metabolic disorder. It is defined as a condition in which the action of insulin, a hormone secreted by the pancreas, is inadequate to keep the blood sugar within what is considered a normal range.

Like all diseases defined by numbers, the level of blood sugar used to make the diagnosis is arbitrary. A fasting blood sugar level—meaning the individual has consumed no calories for at least eight hours—of 126 mg% is considered the threshold for the diagnosis. Similarly, the peak blood sugar after a meal should be less than 180 mg%.

Rather than relying on a blood sugar level at a specific time, the current diagnostic approach is to measure the level of Hemoglobin A1C in blood. This measurement is not affected by meals but rather provides an assessment of the average blood sugar over weeks or months. The test is based on the fact that hemoglobin, a protein in the red blood cell that carries oxygen, becomes coated with sugar in proportion to the average level over time of sugar in the blood. HgbA1C of less than 6.5 percent means blood sugars are consistently in the normal range and diabetes should not be diagnosed. Of course, these arbitrary levels for normal HgbA1C are no better than the arbitrary levels for fasting blood sugar. They are arbitrary.

Diabetes is actually two different diseases, each manifesting the same abnormality in blood sugar. In the so-called juvenile form, or Type 1 diabetes, the pancreas does not produce adequate levels of insulin. This insulin-deficiency syndrome is inherited and usually appears early in life. In the more common adult form, or Type 2, the pancreas produces insulin, but the tissues develop resistance to the effects of insulin. This condition usually develops later in life but is being recognized more often in children these days, presumably because of the increase in childhood obesity.

Both types of diabetes present with elevated blood sugars and increased HgbA1C levels, and both are associated with an increased risk of heart attacks and strokes. But there the similarity ends. Type 1 diabetes is a serious, inherited disease in need of lifetime specialty care. People with Type 1 diabetes are at risk for life-threatening consequences like ketoacidosis, a dramatic metabolic derangement brought on by lack of insulin. Type 2 diabetes also is probably inherited, but its manifestations are very much influenced by diet and weight gain. Its appearance as a disease with elevated blood sugar levels is very much influenced by lifestyle. In Type 2 diabetes, the main concern is not the blood sugar but rather the risk of future cardiovascular disease.

HOW IMPORTANT IS BLOOD SUGAR CONTROL?

Diabetes experts earn their living by controlling blood sugar, which is the standard target in the management of diabetes. New drugs and new devices for monitoring and managing blood sugar levels have flooded the marketplace in recent years. This focus on control of blood sugar or hemoglobin A1C may have deviated the profession from examining the evidence that blood sugar control is that important. This is a story that goes back a long time.

When I was in medical school in the early 1950s, my school taught that blood sugar was not so important as long as the patients received enough insulin to protect them from symptoms and from life-threatening ketoacidosis. A neighboring institution taught just the opposite: rigid control of blood sugar with precisely chosen doses of insulin was critical for the patient's well-being. Sixty years later, we still don't have a clear-cut winner of the argument, despite millions of dollars spent on many carefully designed trials. What has become clear from these studies is that rigid blood sugar control may not be as important as some of the advocates had been preaching.

There is no question that uncontrolled blood sugar can cause symptoms, like thirst and copious urination, and that poorly controlled blood sugar probably increases the risk of infections and may end up damaging the nerves, the kidneys, and the eyes. But the big, life-threatening issue of heart attacks and strokes may not be much influenced by blood sugar control. This is where the large trials have stumbled, usually not showing a significant benefit of therapy aimed at normalizing blood sugar on the risk of heart attacks, strokes, or death. [1]

IS ELEVATED BLOOD SUGAR THE DISEASE?

Since diabetes is diagnosed by an elevation in blood sugar, it is easy to conclude that an elevated blood sugar characterizes the disease. Indeed, a blood sugar of 126 mg% is a prerequisite for the diagnosis, so that arbitrary level may be thought of as representing the disease process. But it never seemed rational to experts to suggest that 125 mg% is normal. By examining data on people with blood sugars from 100 to 125 mg%, epidemiologists concluded that they had a higher risk for cardiovascular disease and death than individuals with blood sugar levels below 100 mg%. Since diabetes experts couldn't call that diabetes, they introduced the term "pre-diabetes," suggesting that such individuals should be advised to alter their lifestyle and be monitored for the possible development of diabetes, that is, a rise in fasting blood sugar to 126 mg% or above.[2]

What is pre-diabetes? From a population standpoint, it could be viewed as a milder form of the disease, since the risk of adverse outcomes is statistically much lower than in those with higher blood sugars. Should it be viewed as a pre-disease state, one in which no treatment is warranted until the blood sugar rises to the diabetes diagnostic range? In other words, is the blood sugar level the disease?

If we view the data on an individual basis, we can reach an alternative conclusion: that diabetes is an abnormal metabolic and cardiovascular state in which blood sugar is higher than ideal but may not necessarily be at the so-called diabetes threshold. It is well known, for example, that some drugs, such as cortisone and other steroid hormones, will lead to the side effect of "diabetes" in some individuals. Recent attention has focused on statin drugs because assessment of the effects of statins in large populations of patients has revealed that taking the medication raises the blood sugar by an average of a few mg%.[3] That rise in blood sugar is considered to be a dangerous side effect of these therapies. Is that true, or did the steroid or the statin merely bring out the abnormal metabolic state in an individual who already had the "disease" but did not yet manifest the elevated blood sugar? Did the steroid place the patient at risk because his or her blood sugar is now elevated, or did the risk already exist in that individual and the blood sugar abnormality was merely precipitated by the steroid or statin drug therapy? Did the rise in blood sugar make the patient a member of the "club" who needs treatment, or was he or she already a member but didn't know it?

The most rational view of pre-diabetes is that some individuals with these borderline higher levels of blood sugar have the disease, diabetes, but have not yet manifested the elevated blood sugar levels. Others in this category are normal. Those with "diabetes" are at heightened risk for cardiovascular disease and should be monitored and, if needed, treated to reduce the risk. Those without "diabetes" need not be placed under heightened scrutiny, at least not for complications of "diabetes." We now know how to assess these individuals for early cardiovascular disease (see chapter 12). Methods certainly exist to challenge these patients metabolically to identify evidence for insulin resistance, but such diagnostic maneuvers have not crept into clinical practice.

HOW DOES DIABETES INCREASE THE RISK FOR CARDIOVASCULAR DISEASE?

Despite the wide acceptance of the relationship between diabetes and atherosclerosis, there is little data to explain the association. One theory, in fact, suggests that they are inherited independently but by closely linked genes that control insulin responsiveness and lipid metabolism. More commonly, experts suspect that something about the metabolic disorder increases the vulnerability of the wall of the artery to infiltration with cholesterol and the formation of plaques.

The most attractive candidate for this interaction is a deficiency in the endothelial secretion and biologic action of nitric oxide. Elevated blood sugars, or perhaps the metabolic derangement that may lead to elevated blood sugars, may impair the secretion and biological activity of nitric oxide, which protects the arterial wall from invasion of lipids and the formation of plaques. It is likely that this abnormality long precedes the rise in blood sugar levels to above 126 mg%. Thus the "disease" leading to cardiovascular morbid events may exist even when blood sugar is in the normal range, and finding those with pre-diabetes who have the "disease" in need of treatment is a useful and potentially life-saving endeavor.

The abnormalities of the small and large arteries represent the "disease," which gets most but certainly not all individuals with diabetes into the "club" of people who need treatment to slow progression of their early cardiovascular disease. Epidemiologists viewing the data recognized that diabetics have on average a similar risk of a first heart attack as nondiabetics with a previous heart attack have of suffering a second heart attack.[4] This is a population-based observation based on statistical risk without any attention to mechanisms. All individuals with a previous heart attack have the "disease," and as members of the "club," they need treatment. Among diabetics, there is a high prevalence of "disease," but many individuals exhibit good cardiovascular health, at least at the time of assessment, and are not members of the "club." As individuals, they should not necessarily be subjected to treatment as if they have the disease, even though they are at high statistical risk because of the metabolic abnormality of "diabetes." They certainly need to be monitored for future membership in the "club."

An inevitable question that arises from this discussion is how much good it does to prevent diabetes from appearing in those with the inherited tendency for insulin resistance. Do the poor dietary and exercise habits that may precipitate an elevated blood sugar in an individual with the underlying disorder make that individual more susceptible to adverse vascular complications? Does the high blood sugar have adverse effects beyond those of the inherited tendency? Perhaps it does. Population statistics support the possibility but really can't address the question. The magnitude of this adverse effect is probably quite small. Individuals who have inherited the diabetic tendency are at risk whether they get fat or not. Complications of "diabetes" are observed in many potentially diabetic patients whose HgbA1C is still normal. So the inherited disorder is a major factor, but a lifestyle that increases blood sugar may play a contributory role.

The likely scenario is that the cardiovascular complications of diabetes relate to the deficiency of nitric oxide, which probably exists long before the blood sugar becomes abnormal in Type 2 diabetes. This deficiency of nitric oxide results in functional and structural abnormalities of the small arteries that adversely affect kidney function; may be associated with nerve pain (neuropathy) in the legs, memory loss, or dementia; and contribute to erectile dysfunction in men. These problems are all more common in diabetics with elevated blood sugars, but they also occur in individuals with sugars below the threshold for diagnosing the disease. They may have inherited the diabetes gene but do not manifest the critical severity of the metabolic component of the disease, perhaps because they have pursued a prudent lifestyle.

Do lifestyle changes have a favorable effect? Exercise improves endothelial function and improves nitric oxide secretion. A fatty meal may worsen endothelial function, and weight loss may improve it. So lifestyle decisions may have an effect on the risk for cardiovascular disease, but the magnitude of this effect is probably overrated by the media and public health authorities. Nonetheless, every little bit helps, and there are many noncardiovascular benefits that accrue from exercise and weight loss.

So the message is clear: pay attention to all the recommendations about diet and exercise. Diabetics need all the help they can get to maintain a healthy cardiovascular system. But their inherited tendency for insulin resistance and nitric oxide deficiency may damage their arteries, and drug therapy aimed at slowing its progression is critical.

WHY IS THE INCIDENCE OF DIABETES RISING?

There is no question that diabetes is more common in American society than it was in the past. Whereas Type 2 diabetes, the kind associated with resistance to the action of insulin, used to be confined predominantly to an older population, the disorder is now appearing more commonly in children and young adults. Have the genes changed or is it the environment?

The metabolic marker for diabetes, the blood sugar, is critically dependent on food intake. If a person has inherited modest insulin resistance but consumes a low-carbohydrate diet, the blood sugar may well remain within the normal range. No diabetes is detected. But if that same individual is addicted to candy bars and eats a dozen a day, the carbohydrate load will undoubtedly overwhelm the insulin control system and result in a rise in blood sugar and an abnormal hemoglobin A1C level. Diabetes is diagnosed.

The genes have stayed the same. Insulin resistance is present, but now dietary indiscretion has precipitated an abnormal blood sugar. Is that elevated blood sugar the culprit in increasing the risk of cardiovascular disease in diabetes, or is it the insulin resistance, which is there with or without an elevated blood sugar? Multiple studies over the years have failed to confirm a robust relationship between lowering blood sugar by diet or drugs and the incidence of heart attacks and strokes. These studies do, however, suggest that kidney disease and eye disease in diabetics are accelerated by poor blood sugar control. For heart attacks and strokes, however, the genetic predisposition to diabetes may be the culprit, not the blood sugar.

So why is the prevalence of diabetes rising in young people? It may not be. What is being observed is an increase in blood sugar because of dietary indiscretion. It is possible that the rising blood sugar may have a subtle accelerating effect on the progression of cardiovascular disease that is initiated by the insulin resistance. But that effect has not yet been documented. Prudence would encourage people with insulin resistance to resist carbohydrate binging, but the warnings about an epidemic of new-onset diabetes are probably misleading.

TREATMENT OF DIABETES

Management of Type 2 diabetes should be aimed primarily at preventing the life-threatening cardiovascular morbid events that threaten all such patients. Although weight loss, exercise, and dietary adjustments are always recommended, it is now well recognized that preventive drug therapy is essential.

The two drug classes that have become essentially mandated therapy for those at risk are statin drugs and inhibitors of the renin-angiotensin system. Statins prevent heart attacks and strokes at least in part by reducing the levels of LDL cholesterol in blood. Angiotensin-converting enzyme inhibitors (ACE) reduce the levels of angiotensin that contribute to blood vessel constriction and to kidney damage that is so common in the diabetic. Drugs in these classes have become standard therapy for diabetics, especially those who are manifesting evidence for cardiovascular disease. As will be emphasized in a subsequent chapter, a prudent approach would be to introduce effective therapy at an earlier stage, once the presence of early disease has been clearly identified, in order to prevent progression of the cardiovascular disease rather than treating after symptoms have developed.

CONTEMPORARY UNDERSTANDING

- Type 1 diabetes is a unique, inherited state of insulin deficiency that requires insulin therapy.
- Type 2 diabetes is a state of insulin resistance that is often accompanied by heightened risk for atherosclerotic morbid events.
- Endothelial dysfunction probably underlies the link between diabetes and cardiovascular disease.
- Diet, exercise, and lifestyle adjustments may modestly delay disease progression, but drug therapy is needed to slow the cardiovascular disease that often accompanies the diabetic state.

- Blood sugar levels may help identify those at heightened risk, but the diabetic state that characterizes this disease process may exist with blood sugar levels below the traditional threshold for its diagnosis.
- Elevated blood sugar is not the disease that threatens life expectancy.

8

SMOKING

CONVENTIONAL WISDOM

- The major risk of smoking is lung cancer.
- Emphysema and chronic lung disease are other serious complications.
- Smoking is dangerous only for the person who smokes.
- Smoking may increase the risk for heart disease, but other factors such as diet and exercise are far more important.
- If you stop smoking, the increased risk disappears.

SMOKING AS A RISK FACTOR

The adverse effects of smoking, especially cigarette smoking, have been widely studied and prominently emphasized over the past few decades. The investigation began with demonstration of the critical relationship between cigarette smoking and lung cancer in the 1950s and 1960s.[1] It was accompanied by clear evidence for causation of bronchitis and emphysema and what has now been labeled as chronic obstructive lung disease or COPD.

The search for lung pathology in individuals who inhaled toxic smoke was a natural association, but the demonstration in more recent years of smoking's contribution to a wide array of diseases outside the lungs, including those of the cardiovascular system, is perhaps more surprising. How does smoking produce so many adverse effects?

ABSORPTION OF TOXINS

The airways in the lungs provide an easily permeable or absorptive surface for substances in inhaled air to get into the bloodstream, where they
circulate throughout the body. We generally think of the stomach and
intestines as a site for absorption of food and drugs that we take by
mouth, but the airways are a source of toxins that we don't necessarily
choose to ingest. Cigarette smoke contains a wide range of substances,
including, of course, nicotine. The effects of nicotine are not due to its
effect on the lungs but rather due to its absorption into the bloodstream.
The other toxic substances in smoke join in by potentially affecting every
organ in the body. The power of these toxic substances becomes apparent
when studying passive smoke inhalation, that smoke we receive uninvited
from a person smoking near us. Strong limitations were placed on smoking in public places, aimed not only at eliminating the unpleasant smell of
cigarette smoke in public areas but also because passive smoke inhalation
exhibits similar patterns of disease occurrence as does active smoking.[2]
Smoking harms more than the smoker.

Smoking increases the rate of occurrence not only of lung cancer but
also of a wide range of other cancers, consistent with the cancer-produc-
ing toxins gaining access to many organs besides the lungs. Smoking also
contributes to a reduction in sperm counts in men, premature delivery in
pregnant women, osteoporosis, cataracts, diabetes, and even rheumatoid
arthritis. The mechanisms of these adverse effects of smoking are not
fully understood, but its effect to produce premature cardiovascular disease may be more understandable.

ENDOTHELIAL DYSFUNCTION

Active and passive smoking may result in damage to the endothelium, or
inner lining, of all the arteries in the body. Damage to endothelial cells
impairs their ability to store or release nitric oxide, which, as previously
described, is needed to relax the artery wall, to inhibit growth of smooth
muscle cells, and to provide a barrier to prevent cholesterol particles from
penetrating the wall of the large arteries to form a plaque of atherosclerosis. When nitric oxide is insufficient, the small artery will constrict, the
walls of both the small and large arteries will thicken from growth of

smooth muscle, plaques will form in the large arteries, and there will be an increased likelihood of clot formation in the arteries, the event that causes myocardial infarctions and strokes.[3] It is no surprise that smoking is associated with a profound increase in the risk of cardiovascular morbid events, including sudden death.

But smoking may also exert its adverse effects by causing oxidative stress. An inadequate nitric oxide effect, classified as endothelial dysfunction, may result from two independent mechanisms. One, as described above, is a reduction in nitric oxide secretion by damaged endothelial cells. The other is the inappropriate inactivation of the secreted nitric oxide gas as soon as it is released. Reactive oxygen species, which can be formed from many chemical reactions, are the prime mechanism of such inactivation.[4] Interest in preserving nitric oxide has led to many efforts to inhibit oxidative stress by administering so-called antioxidants that have become ubiquitous at health food stores. Limited studies of the effectiveness of such interventions have so far failed to find consistent benefit from this intervention.

If you stop smoking, does the increased risk disappear? Many studies have suggested that it does, but their power to determine that is very limited. Smoking accelerates the process of atherosclerosis. This is a chronic process that progresses over time in all of us. Since it is an asymptomatic disease until it results in a morbid event, such as symptoms of coronary artery disease, cerebrovascular disease, or peripheral vascular disease (heart attacks, strokes, or leg cramps when walking), acceleration of the biological process of atherosclerosis is not generally detected until the event takes place. Since smoking accelerates that process, even if one stops smoking and stops the acceleration, the underlying process will be more advanced and disease occurrence as a result of the normal aging process should occur earlier. It is thus far better never to start smoking than to start and then stop.

ARE SOME PEOPLE IMMUNE TO THE SMOKING RISK?

There is no question that individual factors play a strong role in the response to all environmental risk factors. When we opened our cardiovascular disease prevention center in 2000, we wanted to emphasize that our evaluation for early disease was strikingly different from the traditional emphasis on risk factors. We wanted to feature the fact that risk factor assessment provides a statistical estimate of the population risk but not of the presence of disease in an individual. The presence of risk factors, such as smoking, cannot define whether the individual of interest is at risk or not at risk for progression to symptomatic cardiovascular disease. Since our center was focused on keeping people free of cardiovascular disease until age one hundred, we wanted to point out that risk factors themselves are not a reliable determinant. We chose as our "poster girl" the picture of a one-hundred-year-old woman whose family was featured in a *Wall Street Journal* profile. Many of the family had lived into their hundreds, and our "poster girl" was a chain smoker for her entire adult life, so much so that she would not put down her cigarette for the photographer.

Heredity can trump risk factors. Our "poster girl" apparently did not have premature cardiovascular disease, despite her long smoking history. Many other individuals we have studied exhibit extensive cardiovascular disease without any discernible risk factors. The presence of early disease is far more useful for identifying individual risk than all the usual suspects in the environment.

A PUBLIC HEALTH SUCCESS STORY

The dramatic decrease in public smoking in the United States over the past generation is a remarkable success story for public health efforts. A unique combination of health promotion, public fear generation, the distaste of nonsmokers, and the sweeping effect of local laws has succeeded in transforming smoking from a socially attractive activity to one often associated with ostracism.

Efforts to replicate the success of antismoking campaigns with other public health goals have not been nearly as effective. Smoking is a uniquely attractive target. It poisons the atmosphere as well as the individual. Its disappearance improves the quality of life of all, even if it leaves the perpetrator to suffer in silence the pangs of his or her addiction. Nonetheless, the success of community-wide smoking cessation provides an example of how quickly joint action can change behavior.

Yet the adverse effects of smoking have far from disappeared. The sad entertainment industry news in early 2017 was the deaths on subsequent days of actress-writer Carrie Fisher and her mother, movie star Debbie Reynolds. In a documentary on the two, released shortly after their funeral, Carrie is depicted as a heavy smoker whose frequent visits to her mother next door are usually accompanied by a cigarette. Carrie's heart attack and cardiac arrest were likely a consequence of cigarette smoking accelerating her underlying atherosclerotic heart disease. Her mother's death the following day can best be understood as Broken Heart Syndrome, or Takatsubo Syndrome, the stress-induced entity that was described in chapter 2. Smoking harms more than the smoker.

E-CIGARETTES

The escalating interest in e-cigarettes has not yet been accompanied by adequate studies regarding their safety. Indeed, true safety studies of such activities require years of follow-up, which obviously are not yet available. It is hoped by advocates that elimination of the toxins associated with burning will eliminate the non-nicotine adverse effects, including lung cancer and chronic bronchitis and emphysema. Do e-cigarettes cause endothelial damage? The answer is not yet in. Do e-cigarettes increase the likelihood of young people becoming cigarette smokers? That may be the biggest reason to restrict their use.

CONTEMPORARY UNDERSTANDING

- Smoking is dangerous for you and those around you.
- Accelerated cardiovascular disease, especially atherosclerosis, may be a consequence of smoking, but it does not affect all individuals similarly.
- Of all the behavioral activities that may adversely affect the incidence of cardiovascular disease, smoking is by far the most powerful.
- Stopping smoking will reduce the rate of acceleration of cardiovascular disease, but it is unlikely to reverse the abnormalities already produced. Some of its adverse effects probably persist.

9

DIET

CONVENTIONAL WISDOM

- How much you eat is important, but what you eat may be even more important.
- Eating food with saturated fats will cause heart attacks.
- Eating carbohydrates and sweets will cause diabetes.
- Salt is bad for the heart. Never add it to food.
- Adhering to a rigid diet may save your life.
- Everything that tastes good is bad for you.
- You can't be too thin.

THE PUBLIC'S FASCINATION WITH DIETS

No topic has generated as much debate and as many articles and books as the subject of diets. The American public has been fascinated with attempts to adhere to such diets or at least to read about their unique benefits. Vanity has always played a role in our devotion to diets as we focus on our appearance and self-image. But in recent years the emphasis has been on health. Are there diets that promote cardiovascular health and others that impair it?

People generally do not go to their doctor to get a diet plan. Doctors like to give general, nondirective advice. They tend not to be too demanding. Commercial enterprises, however, survive on the basis of more rigid formulas. Books, often written by doctors with a "product" to sell, promote specific foods or specific patterns of consumption, sometimes even calling for specific foods on specific days of the week. So little of this promotional effort has been or can be subjected to careful prospective study of effectiveness that we are largely left with the promoters and detractors free to express themselves without fear of counterevidence.

In early 2016, the Departments of Agriculture and Health and Human Services released their new federal guidelines on diet recommendations.[1] Needless to say it was greeted by the expected controversy, primarily because data are not available to promote or debunk some of the food prejudices favored by certain organizations and corporations. Indeed, some of the rigid rules of the past, like restricting eggs and other cholesterol-containing foods, have been appropriately relaxed. Dietary cholesterol is not the evil we once thought it was. Excess salt is still strongly discouraged, even though salt's danger is probably confined to the subset of individuals who are "salt sensitive" because they cannot fully excrete the salt load. We are approaching the time when the only generally accepted principle will be that people should not get fat.

DIETARY CONTROL OF CHOLESTEROL

Dietary intervention to reduce the risk of atherosclerosis has focused on efforts to lower cholesterol levels, especially that of low density lipoprotein cholesterol (LDL), the "bad" cholesterol that has been associated with the risk of heart attacks and strokes. Initial efforts were to reduce cholesterol in the diet, so eggs became outlawed. Then studies made it clear that preformed cholesterol in the diet has at most a very small effect on cholesterol levels in the body, which are largely related to cholesterol formed by the body. Emphasis thus shifted to reduction of saturated fats and transfats that contribute to the synthesis of cholesterol. Herculean efforts have been made to urge use of polyunsaturated fats, such as margarine and olive oil, to replace butter in the diet. Food manufacturers have marketed "heart healthy" food aimed at limiting cholesterol and saturated fats. Red meats were deemed "dangerous," and consumers were urged to eat fish and chicken. Pork vendors tried to insist that their product was not a "red meat."

But two diets that became very popular were introduced based on the proposition that carbohydrates were the evil, not fats. The Atkins Diet and its disciple, the South Beach Diet, were aimed directly at reducing cardiovascular disease by two cardiologists. They were influenced by the observation that obese and overweight individuals often exhibit elevations of triglycerides, not necessarily cholesterol. This so-called metabolic syndrome was associated with an astoundingly high risk for cardiovascular disease. Since triglycerides are very sensitive to carbohydrate intake, and these individuals often had diets high in "junk" food carbohydrates, their new diets were aimed at dramatic reduction of carbohydrate-containing food products, the Atkins being a rigid reduction and the South Beach more modest. Meat and fats then became acceptable replacements, so the diets directly countered the effort of the American Heart Association and other health agencies to reduce the consumption of red meat.

I recognized early on how individualized was the response to these dietary interventions. I had two patients who decided, not at my urging, to initiate an Atkins Diet. It is not a casual decision because the rigidity of the regimen requires considerable effort, not only for the patient but also for the spouse and family, who usually must share the dietary experience. Both individuals were highly motivated, disciplined, and remarkably attentive to the rules of the diet. Vegetables, breads, and desserts disappeared from their dinner table. Red meats were eaten in abundance. After six months of their dietary discipline, I rechecked their blood levels of cholesterol. In one his LDL cholesterol increased from 155 mg% to 190 mg%, while his triglycerides fell from 275 mg% to 125 mg%, the kind of changes one might expect for people who reduce their carbohydrate but increase red meat consumption.

The other's response was quite astounding. His triglycerides fell dramatically, as expected, from 240 mg% to 90 mg%, but his LDL also fell from an abnormal level of 175 mg% to a normal level of 110 mg%.

The mysteries of individual metabolic variability are not adequately understood to explain these responses, but the experience has convinced me that there is no single diet that will suit everyone and lead to a predictable response. Furthermore, I'm not as sure as many of my colleagues that the LDL increase in the first patient was bad for him or if the reduction in the second patient benefited him. These so-called surrogates for atherosclerosis are not necessarily reliable markers for risk. The disease is in the artery wall, not in the blood where the cholesterol is measured. We need to know if these dietary changes in lipid levels lead to a change in disease progression or in the incidence of morbid events. That kind of data is a lot more difficult to obtain. We know that some drugs that reduce LDL levels also prolong life, but there is no proof that the drug benefit is limited to its effect on LDL levels. No adequately robust study has documented the benefit of dietary lowering of LDL cholesterol.

DIETARY CONTROL OF WEIGHT

The vast majority of diets are aimed at weight loss. Commercial efforts are often augmented by programs that feature counseling and group therapy. The national attention has been directed at the growing prevalence of obesity, and these programs are responding to that perceived need. Although many such programs continue to emphasize the benefits of weight loss on personal appearance and social interaction, health has become an important feature. It is generally accepted that weight loss makes you healthier. Does it?

There is no question that most obese individuals are less healthy than most thin individuals. In particular, cardiovascular disease is more common in obese people, including hypertension and coronary artery disease. Diabetes is certainly more common in obesity. Since obesity is usually accompanied by less physical activity, either as a cause or an effect, the latter may be a contributing factor to the apparent excess of disease. So are we sure that the obesity itself is a cause of disease and its reversal should reduce the risk? Conventional wisdom certainly supports the idea, and our national efforts to rein in obesity are based largely on the conviction that weight loss will improve health.

From an epidemiological standpoint, the hypothesis appears supportable. In large-scale databases, obese individuals have a higher incidence of disease and greater health-care expenditures than thin people.[2] The simple extrapolation from that data is that, if you transform a population from obese to thin, the incidence and cost of disease events will be reduced. But maybe the obese individuals are different. Perhaps their proclivity for obesity is associated with proclivity for disease. Perhaps diet can reduce their obesity but not reverse their proclivity for disease. The only valid test of the hypothesis would be to study a large enough group of obese subjects placed on an effective diet and compare their long-term outcomes with a paired group who do not diet. Small studies seeking to prove the benefits of weight loss have been carried out, but none has succeeded in establishing the benefits of weight loss.

HOW MIGHT OBESITY HARM CARDIOVASCULAR HEALTH

Our old nemesis endothelial dysfunction may be at the root of any adverse cardiovascular health effects of obesity. How does obesity impair nitric oxide activity in the inner lining of the arterial wall? We don't know. It might be inherited and thus not necessarily responsive to diet. It might be related to reduced physical activity level, not to the obesity alone. Otherwise it's not understood how the obesity itself is detected by the endothelium to alter its responsiveness. It could be a substance released by fat cells that affects the endothelial cells. These two structures somehow need to "talk to each other."

Another clear consequence of obesity is that it puts an extra burden on the heart. When an obese patient weighing perhaps 220 pounds walks a half mile, he or she works twice as hard as a 110-pound person. That means twice the oxygen consumption and twice the amount of blood pumped by the heart. It's hardly surprising that heart failure is far more common in obese individuals than in thin ones.[3] Surprisingly, however—and this is called the obesity paradox—obese individuals with heart failure have longer survival than thin people with heart failure.[4]

Like so many risk factors we have considered, it is difficult to prove cause and effect. Proof that reversing the risk factor—in this case, obesity—reduces the extra risk associated with the condition has not been documented. The beauty of drugs that reduce cardiovascular disease morbidity is that they work in everyone, regardless of the mechanisms contributing to the extra risk. So while we seek proof that weight loss improves health, we should recognize that early disease, whatever has accelerated it, can be effectively slowed by drugs aimed at protecting the arteries and heart. Nonetheless, weight loss improves self-perception and quality of life. It's worth accomplishing even if its health benefits are not established.

SALT

Circulating blood contains a good deal of salt or sodium. It is a normal and necessary component of all the fluids in the body. Its concentration in the blood plasma is routinely measured as part of chemical analysis of blood samples. Since the concentration of sodium is closely controlled by adjustment of kidney function, when the body retains extra sodium, it is almost always accompanied by retention of extra water to keep its concentration stable.

So what happens if you down a salty corned beef sandwich with a pickle or if you feast on a batch of salted popcorn, or if you think you are behaving more reasonably and consume a bowl of canned chicken noodle soup? These salt loads are immediately recognized by the body and set up a series of responses. An increase in salt concentration is detected and tells the kidney to retain water to keep the concentration of sodium stable. This immediate expansion of fluid in the system tells the kidney to start eliminating sodium in the urine. These adjustments are delicately managed by secretion of hormones from both the kidney and the brain that can influence kidney function.

In the best of all circumstances, the salt load will be neutralized and eliminated very quickly and nothing else changes. The salt will have no lasting effect. In some individuals, however, perhaps 20 percent of a diverse population but much higher if you study a black population, the hormonal regulatory mechanisms are more sluggish. The salt load is partially reversed, but excess salt and water persist. We label these people as salt sensitive, in contrast to the larger group that we call salt resistant. [5]

In salt sensitive individuals, a high-salt diet raises blood pressure, and this excess salt in the body appears to have an adverse effect on the wall of the arteries, perhaps in part by causing endothelial dysfunction. These individuals should restrict their salt intake. If they have an elevated blood pressure, treatment with a diuretic, which enhances sodium excretion, is highly recommended.

So what about the demand for sodium restriction by health advocacy groups? Is it appropriate? From a population standpoint, restriction of dietary sodium will result in an overall community reduction in blood pressure and presumably a reduction in the community incidence of heart attacks and strokes. It is a good move for the community. But the benefit will be confined to those in the community who are salt sensitive. The others have given up their sodium for no personal gain. Should they be pleased or aggravated?

These comments apply to people who are otherwise healthy. If you have heart failure or kidney disease, the ability of your kidney to excrete salt may be limited by your underlying condition. In those instances, salt restriction may be a necessary component of management.

WHAT DIETARY RULES SHOULD YOU FOLLOW?

Given the individual variability of physiologic responses to what we eat, are there rules that may benefit everyone?

There certainly are principles worth following. Weight gain should be avoided. Although obesity does not adversely affect the arteries and heart in everyone, it increases the risk for endothelial dysfunction and heart enlargement. Maintaining a weight that keeps your BMI well below 30 is at least a first step toward longevity.

Are there foods to be avoided? Not eggs. They are a pretty good source of protein and probably a healthy choice for breakfast. I have friends that avoid egg yolks and order egg white omelets. The yolk in my view is the best tasting part. Carbohydrates should be eaten in moderation. It is their excess that leads to weight gain and a rise in triglycerides. Excess salt should be avoided, especially if your blood pressure is borderline or high or if you suspect you are salt sensitive. Canned soups are an often unsuspected source of salt, and you should check the labeling to seek soups with sodium content of 300–400 mg per portion rather than 600–700 mg.

The diet that appears to come closest to the ideal is the so-called Mediterranean diet. It emphasizes fish, which is an excellent source of healthy protein, but I would have no problem with substituting meat several days a week. The diet emphasizes use of olive oil, but I have no objection to butter now and then. It also advocates nuts, which are a wonderful source of antioxidants and precursors of nitric oxide. Nuts are far and away the best snack to eat, and they should be a part of a good daily diet.

Red wine has always been advocated for its presumed health effects, which makes its benefit on quality of life an added bonus. There has been much attention paid to resveratrol, an antioxidant in red wine that has been identified as the possible mediator of the benefit of red wine on cardiovascular disease. Although this chemical can be administered in pill form, a less pleasant way to seek the benefits of red wine, the data now seems clear that the amount of resveratrol in wine is far too low to account for any health effects. [6]

ARGININE

Arginine is an amino acid that generates nitric oxide (NO) through a biological synthetic process. Arginine is contained in meats, fish, dairy products, grains, and especially nuts. Conventional wisdom suggests that a deficiency of nitric oxide, a first step toward atherosclerosis, is never due to a deficiency of arginine because this amino acid is always present in excess. Nonetheless, arginine is available as a supplement in health food stores. An arginine candy bar has also been marketed. Some investigators have claimed a favorable effect of arginine on blood vessel health. In preliminary studies, my research laboratory has confirmed the possibility that arginine, taken in adequate quantities as a supplement, can favorably affect the function of small arteries. [7]

Definitive studies of the effectiveness of arginine in reducing the progression of cardiovascular disease have not been conducted. Such studies would be very expensive. Private corporations are unlikely to conclude that the cost of such a study, if successful, could be offset by sales of arginine, which is cheap to manufacture and sell. Nonetheless, I have encouraged some individuals, whose disease appears to be progressing despite standard therapy, to initiate arginine supplement therapy. Anecdotal experience is encouraging.

CONTEMPORARY UNDERSTANDING

- Obesity identifies individuals with a higher risk for cardiovascular disease.
- The mechanism of this increased risk is not fully understood.
- There are many good reasons to prevent or reverse obesity, but prevention of cardiovascular disease can be only a conjectural one.

- Unique dietary regimens may be an effective tool to encourage weight loss, but eating less and exercising more are the most effective strategies.
- Eating a fatty diet does not necessarily raise your bad cholesterol level, and eating too much carbohydrate certainly can adversely affect the fat levels in your blood.
- Diet is not the major factor in determining the cholesterol levels in your blood.
- Salt has adverse cardiovascular effects in a sizable minority of the population, but it is well tolerated by most.
- Nuts probably benefit cardiovascular health.

10

INFLAMMATION

CONVENTIONAL WISDOM

- Infections, arthritis, and cancers are diseases that have nothing to do with the cardiovascular system.
- If you successfully treat these diseases, the patient need not worry about other problems.
- Heart disease is caused by other unrelated mechanisms.

INFLAMMATION AND CARDIOVASCULAR DISEASE

In recent years, it has become apparent, after examining large clinical databases, that a number of medical diseases not directly affecting the heart or blood vessels are associated with an excess risk for cardiovascular disease, especially coronary artery disease. Such an association always requires great scrutiny before one can conclude that there is a mechanistic relationship. Such associations may coexist just because the diseases are common. Perhaps the presence of one has led caregivers to search for the other.

The association appears to be particularly strong with diseases characterized as "inflammatory." These diseases activate the immune system, which calls forth a response to attack the invader, such as a bacterium. In chronic diseases, however, inflammation can result from autoimmunity, that mistake of nature that tells the individual's immune system that a normal tissue is an "invader." Most of these diseases exhibit a chronic inflammatory component; that is, they stimulate the body's immune response. Rheumatoid arthritis is a good example. The normal joint tissue is viewed by the body's immune system as a foreign invader. The inflammatory response gradually destroys the joint tissue and the joint. Atherosclerosis also appears to exhibit an inflammatory component.

Why do inflammatory diseases like rheumatoid arthritis increase the risk for atherosclerosis?

HOW DOES INFLAMMATION AFFECT VASCULAR FUNCTION AND STRUCTURE?

The formation of cholesterol plaques on the arterial wall is an inflammatory process that activates antibodies and immune cells. In recent years, it has become apparent that individuals with accelerated atherosclerosis demonstrate elevated levels of inflammatory markers, such as C–reactive protein or CRP, thus confirming that the process in the artery wall has an inflammatory component to it. The endothelial cells of the inner lining of all arteries are very sensitive to this inflammatory process. It is likely that activation of the immune system impairs the function of these endothelial cells and reduces the synthesis and availability of nitric oxide that protects the inner surface of the blood vessel wall. This effect makes the wall more vulnerable to deposits of cholesterol and more vulnerable to aggregation of platelets that induce clots. Thus inflammation appears to be a mechanism of inducing heart attacks and strokes. [1]

The prominence of inflammation in coronary artery plaques led to an interest in determining if C-reactive protein (CRP), a blood marker for the inflammatory process, is elevated in patients with coronary disease. Indeed, some enthusiasts claimed that CRP should be added to standard risk markers in identifying the risk for a future heart attack. [2] It turns out that CRP may be slightly higher in patients with coronary artery disease than in those without, but the magnitude of the association is very small and it turns out to be a pretty insensitive measurement. Although we do measure CRP as one of the standard laboratory tests in our assessment of an individual's cardiovascular health, I find it of little value and do not advocate its measurement to help identify an individual's risk.

WHAT ARE THE INFLAMMATORY DISEASES?

Several common diseases have been demonstrated to accelerate atherosclerosis. The most recent is HIV-AIDS, which has been transformed by drug therapy from a lethal to a chronic disease process. Whereas AIDS patients formerly died of their HIV virus, they are now more commonly dying much later from atherosclerotic disease.[3] Whether acceleration of the atherosclerosis is caused by the virus, its treatment, or the accompanying inflammation is uncertain, but the association is real.

Cancer survivors are another large group now susceptible to accelerated atherosclerosis. It is unclear if their apparent endothelial dysfunction is caused by the inflammatory tumor or by the chemotherapy used to obliterate it, but the risk for premature atherosclerosis is definitely increased in cancer survivors.

Rheumatoid arthritis is another common disease in which chronic inflammation, in this instance in the joints of the body, exists for years. Such individuals exhibit a strikingly increased risk for heart attacks and strokes, clear evidence for accelerated atherosclerosis.[4]

As far as we know, these inflammatory-induced causes of atherosclerosis can be slowed by drugs that are effective in slowing the atherosclerotic process in individuals without these diseases. So treatment should be the same as in other individuals who have joined the "club" in need of treatment. It is not necessary to understand all the causes of atherosclerosis in order to treat the biological process.

The idea that anti-inflammatory drugs could be effective in countering the progression of atherosclerosis has been vigorously pursued. Studies with various anti-inflammatory agents have so far failed to document a favorable effect on the atherosclerotic process.[5] Perhaps the right agent hasn't yet been studied. Perhaps the studies have been inadequate to document a benefit. Additional studies are in progress. For the moment, treatment with statins, renin-angiotensin inhibitors, and other antihypertensive drugs is the most effective strategy.

Are all patients with rheumatoid arthritis members of the "club" in need of cardiovascular preventive therapy? No. The incidence is higher and justifies investigation, but the prevalence of disease is not high enough to accept all such individuals into the "club."

CONTEMPORARY UNDERSTANDING

- Atherosclerosis is an inflammatory process.
- Diseases that involve chronic inflammation increase the likelihood that atherosclerosis will progress and lead to complications, such as heart attacks and strokes.
- C-reactive protein measurement is not very useful in identifying the atherosclerotic process.
- Treatment aimed at the inflammation has not yet proved to be effective.

11

STATISTICS VERSUS BIOLOGY

CONVENTIONAL WISDOM

- The most reliable medical knowledge comes from large populations in whom statistical tests of significance determine optimal treatment.
- Risk factors for disease are identified by correlations carried out in large populations of patients.
- Effectiveness of therapy can only be documented by tests in a large population that demonstrate significant benefit.
- Guidelines for medical management are dependent for their recommendations on tests of significance in large populations.
- Although understanding the biologic process of disease is an important asset for health-care providers, decisions about diagnosis and treatment are dependent on rigid criteria for diagnosis and treatment that are based on statistical analysis.
- The era when doctors used their judgment rather than guidelines is over.

A GENERATIONAL SHIFT

The past generation has witnessed a remarkable shift in the way disease is diagnosed and treated. When I went to medical school and began practicing medicine in the mid-1950s, the diagnosis and management of disease was often viewed as an art form. Thinking through a constellation of symptoms and physical findings was a challenge to physicians, and the successful ones became labeled as diagnosticians. It was an intellectual challenge that favored those with experience and a prepared brain. Students and trainees flocked to their sides to hopefully learn some of their magical insights. The medical literature was rich with case studies— observations on individual patients who presented with unique findings, unique diagnoses, or remarkable responses to new therapy. Medical education was dependent on learning the intricacies of diagnosis and treatment from master physicians.

In the past few decades, all that has changed, and most experts now believe that the change is for the better. Rather than isolated islands of presumed excellence, the professional view that emerged was that what we needed were standards of care available to everyone, not just the disciples of the great physicians. We could no longer rely on unique insights of a fertile mind. We needed documentation, clear-cut rules for diagnosis, and studies of therapeutic responses that met rigorous statistical criteria. It was time, medical experts opined, to move medicine from an art form to a science.

This transition has changed the hierarchy in medical practice. The physician, with his or her store of knowledge and judgment, always had served as the leader in a health-care environment. That changed. Doctors have gradually and largely become subservient to the system, a system of health care organized not only to standardize care but to generate the maximum possible revenue with the minimum time spent on patient care. Of course, this shift was a consequence of the change in medical funding from an unstated contract between the patient and the provider to a more complex contract between the provider's organization and the patient's insurance carrier. But the transition from art form to science made this contractual arrangement possible. Since doctors were supposedly all "playing from the same playbook," all doctors could be considered equal. The eminent diagnostician has lost his cachet. A fee structure can now be applied to all caregivers. This has discouraged the kind of interaction that in the past served as the basis of the doctor-patient relationship. It has also standardized the management of illnesses that may in the past have been treated creatively but often inadequately.

Health-care providers were in the past given remarkable freedom. Contemplation about a patient's symptoms could lead to an unusual and unapproved management strategy that the prescriber conjured up out of his or her own experience and insight. The management was creative, and it might have been remarkably effective or woefully inappropriate. No board oversaw this management strategy, and there was no threat to reimbursement. The marketplace tended to reward successful doctors and penalize the failures. Are we better off today with more regimented diagnoses and management? Some would say yes and others no.

With this new system of health care, leadership shifted from the doctor to the administrator, the financial officer, and the biostatistician. Data became power, and analysis of data, similar to that of retailers or food chains, became the driving force in health care. Biology as the focus of health care has been replaced by statistics.

An analogy might be the desire to form a basketball team. A statistician reviewing data might appropriately conclude that the best basketball players are over 6 feet 5 inches tall. He or she might then proceed to select for the team all people over that height. The statistician is correct on the basis of likelihood but woefully deficient on the basis of musculoskeletal ability. A few minutes evaluating the skill of individuals would exclude many of the tall candidates and identify the talent of many of the shorter ones. Statistics should never completely replace judgment.

MAKING A DIAGNOSIS

In the middle of the twentieth century, a diagnosis was often the goal of health care. Doctors constructed long lists of so-called differential diagnoses to consider and work through over time and often subsequent visits. Understanding the disease, far more important than a specific diagnostic term, was the target for the caring physician. A diagnosis was important, but care could be given while possible diagnostic categories were being considered.

That focus on biology and on understanding the disease has been diminished in the current health-care system. A diagnosis is now essential because that is how doctors and clinics and hospitals bill for their service. Not having a diagnosis is tantamount to not seeing the patient. And that diagnosis must match the official list of diagnostic codes now having evolved into a list called the ICD-10, which stands for International Classification of Disease, Revision 10. The ICD-10 now rules the world of reimbursement.

There is nothing wrong with expecting a caregiver to provide a diagnosis for a patient visit. Flexibility in how the doctor labels a visit would seem to be essential. Suppose a slightly elevated blood pressure was recorded on a first visit. The provider is hesitant to label the patient as "hypertension" since that diagnosis might have implications for such things as health insurance. So he or she might want to use a slightly different term in order to get reimbursed for the visit. But the ICD-10 is rigid about what the disorder is called. Furthermore, there is a long list of diagnostic codes for hypertension from which the caregiver must select one. Is this long list appropriate because of important differences that can be useful in understanding the disease and its ramifications? For the most part, the amazingly long list of diagnostic codes has little to do with biology or with the understanding of the disease process. It is aimed at putting the patient into a box that the coders thought would characterize a disease process, but which in fact largely leads to arbitrary decisions that have little to do with the actual disease process. It is part of the current generation's insistence that all the lines on a form be completed even if they contribute nothing to an understanding of the disorder for which the patient came to see the caregiver. It provides health-care systems and insurance companies with data from which observations about health care are promulgated. The reliability of such data is less certain.

TREATING A PATIENT

Fifty years ago doctors initiated specific therapy for illnesses based on their personal experience and on publications in respected journals. Treatment was not uniform. Some experts used drugs with which primary care providers might be unfamiliar. Some physicians persisted in using therapy that had been discredited by journal articles. If there was a correct treatment, but not everyone was being given it, the quality of health care was being harmed by this variability.

The new, more organized health-care system began developing guidelines. These guidelines were not only designed to elevate and standardize health care throughout the country, but they also began spawning efforts to promote "standards of care." When a therapy or procedure had been established by large-scale studies in large populations to be effective in treating a disease, especially if it turned out to be life-saving, then it could be used as a measure of an institution's or a clinic's quality of care. If mammography, for instance, was determined to be a critical test for women of a certain age, then the fraction of women of that age in any health-care system who were referred for mammography could be used as a measure of that clinic's quality of care. If such measures become a factor in reimbursement, then it might become a top priority of a health-care administrator. Such efforts may distort the traditional doctor-patient relationship and lead to a focus on things that may not be so important but are revenue sources.

So in the new health-care system, the diagnosis is key to the treatment strategy. In the old days, a doctor evaluated patients individually and tried to make judgments reflecting a comprehensive understanding of the patient, the biology of their disease, and how any specific therapy might influence their quality and duration of life. The ability of the health-care provider to make that assessment, and the reliability of any such assessment, could never be established. So the system changed. Now the diagnosis, rigidly defined by the ICD-10 code,[1] leads to a guideline for treatment that may recommend a therapy for which its use is viewed as a standard of care. Not prescribing it becomes a burden to the doctor, who must now explain in the medical record why it is not being employed. And failure to use this "standard of care" may adversely affect the clinic's reimbursement. It is easier for the doctor to follow the prescribed path, even if his intuition is that the specific therapy may not be right for the specific patient. It worked in a large population, the guidelines say, and your patient has the same diagnosis, so it should work in your patient, too. This argument is, of course, fallacious. But there is no way to prove your patient is an outlier. Biology and intuition are not substitutes for statistics in the current health-care system.

MECHANISM OF DISEASE

Illnesses in need of diagnosis and treatment do not necessarily come in neat packages that match ICD-10 codes. Illnesses are biological processes in which physiological systems may be altered. Body temperature rises and one has fever due to a wide range of inflammatory disturbances. Blood pressure may rise or fall due to a physiological alteration in the arteries or the heart, which determine blood pressure. A joint may swell because of altered physiology in the joint itself. A headache may develop because of a wide range of disturbances that affect the pain fibers to the head or scalp. The challenge to the health-care provider is to understand these physiological processes, to sort out all the potential disturbances to normal physiology, and to select the one or ones that may be playing a role in this particular patient. Although statistical likelihoods always play a role in the diagnostic process, the ultimate diagnosis will be more influenced by history, physical findings, and the judgment of the caregiver. Finding a diagnostic code to facilitate categorization and billing can work against the effort to understand the patient's problem.

Unfortunately the current health-care system does not encourage contemplation and the understanding of mechanisms of disease. By demanding use of ICD codes and guidelines for management and by limiting patient visits to fifteen or twenty minutes, the health-care system has greatly curtailed the freedom of the health-care provider to contemplate.

GUIDELINES

Management of disease is now largely driven by guidelines.[2] These guidelines recommend treatment strategies for individuals with diseases defined by ICD codes. The guidelines are developed by expert panels of caregivers with expertise in the specific field of the disease process. But the panel does not make its recommendations based on the personal expertise of the individual members but rather usually by reviewing the results of carefully performed clinical trials designed to objectively assess the effectiveness of various alternate therapies. The gold standard for this evaluation is carefully designed clinical trials demanding rigorous statistical evidence for the benefit of specific forms of therapy.

Clinical trials of this type are an example of population medicine. Patients are selected to participate in such trials if they meet rigorous entrance criteria. It may be a blood pressure above a certain arbitrary level, such as 140/90 mmHg. It may be a blood cholesterol value above some arbitrary level. These may be the same criteria used for ICD-10 code diagnoses. The protocol may list a number of other entrance requirements and a number of exclusions in order to capture the specific population the study is designed to investigate.

Studies may be short-term, such as blood pressure lowering, or long-term when the study seeks to address morbid events or life expectancy. But the goal of any clinical trial is to establish if the population selected for the study exhibits a statistically significant benefit of the therapy being tested. The patients entered into the study are all individuals who shared at least one criterion—an elevated blood pressure or an elevated cholesterol—but there their similarity ceases. Their mechanism of disease may have been entirely different. They are hereditarily and environmentally different from each other. A statistically significant benefit of a single treatment strategy in the overall population does not imply that everyone in the population benefited similarly. But the study is taken to document the benefit of the treatment. The guideline committee is obligated to state the benefit. The health-care system embraces the guidelines. In an ideal world, the establishment contends, everyone will be treated with the beneficial agent.

We have served the population but not necessarily the individual. Is there a way to document individual responsiveness in an objective manner?

THE "N OF 1" EXPERIMENT

Advertisements for various procedures, supplements, and medications include testimonials from individuals who proclaim benefit on their health. We all know the fallibility of these compliments. They are uncontrolled observations compounded by the personal bias of the spokesperson. The compliments are also hand-picked by the sponsor from perhaps other less-enthusiastic statements. These testimonials have no credence.

We also are exposed to comments by friends and acquaintances who may extol the virtues of various interventions they have come to appreciate. We may respect the desire of these friends to be helpful, but we recognize that their advocacy does not mean that the treatment is effective or that it will favorably affect another individual. These are all uncontrolled observations by biased observers.

Is there a way to obtain unbiased evidence on an individual's response to a treatment? Can we move from the rigor of population response in a clinical trial to unbiased individual response?

The only option is an "n of 1" experiment, meaning an experiment on one person. I will describe such an experiment that I conducted some years ago on a man with severe heart failure, a manifestation of advanced heart disease with a shortened life expectancy.

The patient was hospitalized and not responding to our usual therapy, which at the time in 1970 was very limited. I decided, based on my attempts to understand the biologic process from which he suffered, to start treatment with an old drug that I thought might unburden his heart by relaxing the arteries, not by affecting the heart directly. He got remarkably better and went home taking the drug in frequent doses around the clock. No other studies had been undertaken with this drug, so my treatment was certainly not advocated or being used by others.

I would see the patient in my clinic at regular intervals. He continued to do well, and he and his wife were delighted to maintain the regimen, which included doses of the drug in the middle of the night. After some months of this management, I saw him in clinic one day with a new medical resident who was skeptical of the benefit. Since there was no literature supporting my approach, he questioned whether the response was anything but a biased observation. He suggested that the patient had gotten better through no act of mine, but he had attributed the benefit to a drug that I, as his physician, was enthusiastic about. He frankly didn't believe the drug was effective, and he convinced me to document it.

I undertook a study that today would have been ethically unthinkable. Without the patient's or his wife's consent, I substituted a placebo or dummy medication for the drug I had been giving him. The intent was to make certain the patient was unaware the drug had been stopped. If I had just withdrawn the pill, he would have known and perhaps been influenced by that knowledge. This was a true blinded experiment. The treatment had been discontinued, but the patient did not know.

Three days later I had a frantic call from his wife. He was back in severe heart failure, unable to breathe, sweating, and near death. Emergent reintroduction of his therapy restored him to his previous state. The experiment worked, but we almost lost the patient. The therapy was effective.

But such "n of 1" experiments are not adequate to approve a therapy for anyone but the individual in the study.[3] Do all patients benefit or only this one? Are there risks and side effects that may limit its effectiveness? What fraction of a population with this disease will benefit? The FDA could never approve a drug for treatment based on a study of a single individual.

Years passed after this observation in 1970 before this drug and drugs like it were approved for treatment of heart failure. During those years, I used these drugs to treat scores of patients who I think had an improved quality of life and, as subsequently demonstrated, an improved duration of life. I was using an understanding of pathophysiology and clinical experience to benefit my patients. Such innovation is no longer encouraged in the current health-care system.

Unfortunately there is no middle ground. Clinical trials in populations and "n of 1" experiments in an individual leave a vast area of uncertainty. How can we devise therapies for individuals without more knowledge? Can genomic studies bridge the gap? No. They are really population data with statistical likelihoods based on genes rather than on eligibility criteria. They move us only a little closer to individualized medicine. Our tools are limited. We are misguiding the public if we don't admit it.

A SOLUTION TO THE DILEMMA

Not knowing how to treat an individual patient because he or she may not respond the same way that a large population on average responded represents a dilemma. Guidelines provide no advice. Doctors are left with uncertainty, usually accepting the mean response in clinical trials as the guide to treatment. Individual patients are assumed to be representative of the clinical trial population, based only on some similarity of the criteria used to recruit patients into the trial. Their individual characteristics and, more importantly, their heredity and their potentially unique mechanisms of disease cannot be considered.

But there is a potential way out of this dilemma. Therapies based on guideline recommendations are designed to meet at least one of two goals: make the patient feel better or make the patient live longer. All of medical therapy is designed to meet one, the other, or both of these goals. If your treatment doesn't make the patient feel better (physically or psychologically) or make him or her live longer, the treatment is not effective.

It would seem simple to evaluate the "feel better" criterion. Just observe the patient or ask the patient whether the treatment has relieved symptoms or improved well-being. That would be fine if observations made by the patient or the caregiver were objective, but in fact they are so influenced by potential bias that their reliability is seriously flawed. The "n of 1" experiment described above is a formal way to remove bias, but use of this design in everyday practice isn't easily accomplished. So the "feel better" criterion cannot be promoted as an anticipated response in others with the same condition. The FDA cannot accept such potentially biased data as evidence of a therapeutic response. But making the patient feel better is one goal of treatment. If this patient feels better, even if it is only their perception of relief, the treatment was successful, at least for now.

The goal of life prolongation only applies to conditions that are life-threatening. High blood pressure and high cholesterol call for treatment not because of symptoms but because of the threat for premature death. As noted earlier, the FDA has allowed blood-pressure reduction and cholesterol reduction to be a target for therapy with drugs that have been approved for that indication. But there is a growing demand for the drugs also to exhibit a benefit on survival, especially because they have no benefit on symptoms that are not usually present in such patients. Here is where increasingly large trials with many thousands of patients are required. Are we obligated to accept the large trial evidence of a statistically significant reduction in mortality as a guide to the benefit of therapy in an individual? Does the population of individuals selected for participation in a clinical trial provide adequate evidence for management of the individual in the doctor's office?

Can the caregiver inform the patient that the clinical trial evidence and guidelines for therapy should assure him or her that the therapy being prescribed is life-prolonging? Furthermore, can the patient be appropriately advised that the therapy for blood pressure and cholesterol should be continued for the rest of the patient's now longer life?

I have always been troubled by the long-term trial design requirement that patients be followed until enough of them die to document that treatment has led to a significant reduction in mortality rate. Why wait until people die to document that the treatment was a failure? Death is not a random event. In most of the cardiovascular diseases we study, death is a consequence of progression of artery or heart disease. Why don't we monitor progression of disease to determine if our treatment is adequately slowing it? We now can assess disease progression using noninvasive tests. Can we use disease progression as a substitute for mortality to document the effectiveness of therapeutic interventions?

Despite the attractiveness of this strategy, the health-care forces oppose it. The FDA insists that its mandate is to document a survival benefit and refuses to accept measures of disease progression as a surrogate for mortality. Guideline developers insist that large clinical trials can never adequately assess mechanisms of disease and its progression. Such observations, they claim, may be grossly misleading. They are right, of course, if the wrong markers for disease progression are selected, or if the approach under study exerts some noncardiovascular effect that shortens life.

But the reliability of measures of cardiovascular function and structure that underlie disease progression should be subjected to careful study and validation. Rather than rejecting the concept of disease progression as a surrogate for morbidity and mortality, the health-care establishment should undertake definitive studies in an attempt to find an alternative to impossibly large trials designed to document mortality reductions from new approaches to treatment.

Documentation of the benefit of a therapy to reduce the risk of getting sick or dying in asymptomatic individuals, who have a very low event rate over reasonable durations of monitoring, will be particularly difficult. If our goal is to devise optimal therapy to extend healthy life expectancy, it is essential that we devise reliable methodology to track progression of disease and to demonstrate the favorable effect of therapy on that progression. It is critical that this effort be successful.

CONTEMPORARY UNDERSTANDING

- Statistical analysis of population data informs health-care providers about likelihood of therapeutic effectiveness but cannot be the sole driver of individual management.
- Effectiveness and safety of interventions may vary widely among different individuals in any population.
- Guidelines are useful in establishing principles of management but should not mandate therapy in everyone.
- The process of selecting treatment for individuals should be informed by statistical analysis of populations, but individualized treatment re-

quires an understanding of the biological disease process and the mechanisms of treatments that may interfere with progression of the individual's disease process.

12

DETECTION OF EARLY DISEASE

CONVENTIONAL WISDOM

- Cardiovascular disease can be recognized in asymptomatic individuals, but the diagnostic process is costly and should not be routinely undertaken.
- The search for early disease may uncover unexpected abnormalities that need not be treated.
- Healthy people without symptoms should be left alone and not subjected to diagnostic tests and unnecessary therapy.
- Lifestyle changes are good for everyone, but only people with high blood pressure and high cholesterol levels are known to be at high risk and only they should be treated with drugs.
- Assessment of risk factors and calculation of statistical risk for cardiovascular disease, based on standard screening tests, is the only diagnostic tool necessary to determine what, if anything, should be done for an asymptomatic adult.

POPULATION VS. INDIVIDUAL RISK

Cardiovascular disease will disable or kill about half of American men and women. It is not surprising, therefore, that care for patients with cardiovascular disease is far and away the largest contributor to health-care costs, reaching an estimated expenditure of over a trillion dollars per year in the United States.[1] That cost, plus the cost to society of the shortened symptom-free life of so many of our residents, should stimulate the country to do something about it. But the public underestimates what can be done. They seem to think that these morbid events are inevitable, even if they could be slightly delayed, and that there is no solution to the costs except making management of the events more efficient.

The public health agencies of our country have approached the problem as a population issue. We are growingly obese and growingly sedentary, characteristics that we know are statistically associated with an increase in prevalence of disease. Therefore, health agencies promote efforts starting in childhood to educate the population to eat more prudently and exercise more. The aim of this effort seems appropriate. Unsavory behavior patterns may result in excess risk, so reduce the excess risk. But this approach disregards the "elephant in the room." It goes for the "low-hanging fruit." Yes, behaviors that may raise blood pressure, increase waist circumference, and even raise cholesterol and triglyceride levels likely increase the risk of cardiovascular disease, but that increase is only modest. If blood pressure and cholesterol rise above our arbitrary thresholds of "abnormal," then treatment may appropriately be initiated. This approach leaves most high-risk individuals untreated. Even if a healthy lifestyle keeps the blood pressure and cholesterol and waist circumference within a "healthy" range, early cardiovascular disease may be lurking. The conventional approach disregards the fact that most of the individual risk is not contained in obesity and inactivity or in any other risk factor. Reliance on a poor lifestyle and on arbitrary levels of risk factors to recommend intervention leaves most of the at-risk population undetected and untreated.

This individual risk is largely inherited through a person's genomic makeup. A useful analogy is to view cardiovascular health as a car driving down a highway—the highway of life—that ends in a lethal cardiovascular morbid event, perhaps preceded by little accidents along the way. Every car will eventually reach an accident—the nonfatal morbid event or the lethal end of the road—unless it is destroyed by some other noncardiovascular fatal event along the way. But the speed of the car—the rate of aging and disease development in the arteries and heart—is what determines how long it takes to get to the end of the road. If the car slows enough, noncardiovascular events, such as cancer or automobile accidents, may terminate the trip before the end of the road. The rate of the car is largely set in the genes and inherited characteristics. Certain behavior patterns can alter the speed by "stepping on the accelerator." For Carrie Fisher, as noted in chapter 8, it was cigarette smoking. Diet and exercise and other healthy activities can take the foot off the gas pedal. But appropriately administered drugs—pharmacotherapy—can apply the brakes. We already have effective drugs if individually and properly administered, and I am confident we will develop even more effective pharmacologic agents in the near future. These are needed to "apply the brakes." But they must be administered selectively and specifically to those whose disease is progressing too rapidly for them to reach a healthy advanced age.

It mystifies me why so many people shun the idea of taking drugs to "slow the car." They willingly submit themselves for cancer detection and take antibiotics for infection, but the idea of drug therapy to slow progression of cardiovascular disease is anathema to many. Perhaps they think the recommendation for preventive drug therapy is a subversive plot by the pharmaceutical industry to sell more pills. But it isn't. The medication currently used to slow progression is all generic. The pills are cheap and should be free. Industry has shown no enthusiasm for marketing preventive therapy. And doctors tend to think of it as a "last resort," when lifestyle adjustments are inadequate to lower a raised blood pressure or an elevated cholesterol level. We aren't paying enough attention to the speeding car, until an accident gets our attention or premature death gains our sympathy. When was Antonin Scalia told he had early disease in need of treatment? Was he aware he had joined the "club"? Or was his sudden death a surprise to all? Regardless of your view about his voting record on the Supreme Court, his car reached the end of the road before it should have.

Instead of advocating for early disease detection and drug intervention to slow its progression, health authorities have focused on lifestyle choices as the cause of disease and as the solution to the problem.[2] The pervasiveness of this message is out of proportion to the meager evidence for its validity. Yes, there is an association between markers purported to be associated with poor lifestyle choices and the severity of cardiovascular disease, and we all want to believe that correcting the lifestyle will reduce the risk of advanced disease. But, as we have emphasized before, association does not necessarily mean cause-and-effect. Cause-and-effect requires documenting that altering the lifestyle favorably affects the disease process. The failure of most clinical trials to demonstrate the benefits of such interventions has encouraged a robust search through data bases to document a benefit from prudent lifestyle choices. The most recent and impressive effort was published in December 2016 in the *New England Journal of Medicine*.[3] The investigators analyzed data from more than 55,000 individuals who participated in long-term cardiovascular disease outcome studies. They classified them by DNA analysis into three hereditary risk groups, based solely on the presence or absence of genetic markers that have appeared in prior studies to track with the likelihood of coronary artery disease. They confirmed that these DNA subgroups identified populations with different risk, thus confirming that heredity plays an important role in determining future cardiovascular disease. They then examined what they identified as lifestyle choices that they assumed were independent of DNA. These included smoking, obesity, exercise and diet—markers for health that may actually be greatly influenced by unknown genetic factors. Yes, these markers exert influence on their genetic risk, and the data on smoking as a disease contributor is most robust. But the genetic determinants of these apparent lifestyle choices remain unexamined. This association can never substitute for a definitive study documenting that alterations in lifestyle can prevent cardiovascular disease morbid events. Such documentation is still largely deficient. Is it okay to stress to the public the virtue of a prudent lifestyle? Probably yes. Is it okay to suggest to the public that this is the way to prevent heart disease? Probably not, in the absence of documentation.

PROGRESSION OF DISEASE

Cardiovascular morbid events—heart attacks, strokes, heart failure, vascular obstruction in the legs and kidneys, etc.—are all preceded by years of progression of measurable disease in the arteries or heart. Even young Egyptian mummies had measurable disease in their arteries and hearts. A recent discovery was a 5,300-year-old Tyrolean iceman who had extensive calcification of atherosclerotic plaques in his coronary arteries.[4] Moderate slowing of the disease's progression, which is the best diet and exercise can do, will at best produce only a small reduction or delay in future morbid events. These lifestyle changes might produce a slight downtrend in the event rates in a society or community, a numerical decline that might make the health-care agencies feel fulfilled. But preventable events will still keep occurring in individuals who are often thin and active and have none of the features that would lead them to be identified for treatment. Furthermore, by attempting to impose these population efforts on everyone—even those without any measurable early disease who will never suffer from such an event—the agencies are sacrificing many people's individual preferences to benefit the society. We should be more discriminating than that.

The medical profession uses a guide to who is at risk for cardiovascular disease, not by searching for early disease likely to progress, but by applying population data obtained by knowing the individual's age, gender, height, and weight and by measuring blood pressure and cholesterol levels. Since increments in these "risk factors" are associated with increments in the population incidence of cardiovascular morbid events, epidemiologists and biostatisticians have convinced the medical profession that these are the variables that need to be treated in individual patients. These experts fail to accept the modesty of the relationship between these variables and the events. They are statistically associated, but they are not powerful determinants of individual risk.

One of the weaknesses of most statistical attempts to calculate risk is that the risk is often assessed at ten years. Therefore, treatment recommendations are often made on the basis of an elevated ten-year risk for developing a morbid event. But our population is growingly concerned about long-term or lifetime risk. If I'm forty years old, my concern may not be a heart attack in the next ten years but one occurring at thirty, forty, or even fifty years. Our outlook is increasingly long-term. I'd like never to suffer from a cardiovascular morbid event. At our prevention center, our aim is to keep people free of cardiovascular disease through the age of one hundred. I try to convince all my patients that we know how to identify early disease, we know how to treat it to prevent its progression, and we therefore know potentially how to keep them healthy from a cardiovascular standpoint until they have completed a century of life. The earlier we can identify the disease, of course, the more likely will be the substantial prolongation of life.

Those individuals with very early disease are likely to have a very low ten-year risk. If surviving for ten years without a morbid event is the measuring stick for low risk, one misses entirely the forty-year-old whose disease is progressing during those ten years and is on track for a heart attack at age sixty. Therapy introduced at age forty could slow progression and add years to his life, but the medical establishment discourages any attempt to identify that early disease in need of treatment. Conventional thinking is harming cardiovascular health.

HOW WE IDENTIFY EARLY DISEASE

The vast majority of morbid events result from progression of disease in the arteries or heart, the kind of disease described in chapter 1. Some of these morbid events result from blockages in the large arteries that deprive organs and tissues of nourishment from blood supply. Some result from narrowing of small arteries that limit nourishment of small regions of the tissues. Some result from damage or disruption of the heart muscle or heart valves that impairs the heart's pump function or destabilizes the heart rhythm. All of these events are a consequence of long-term progression of these abnormalities, and all of them can be detected and treated. This progression is not over weeks or months but over years.

The changes in cardiovascular function or structure that characterize this early disease can now be detected by simple tests of function or by imaging techniques that have become readily available in recent years. Some of the imaging methods, such as CAT scans, involve radiation exposure, and some, like magnetic resonance imaging (MRI), require expensive equipment and large centers. These techniques are aimed at specific organs, usually the heart, and can detect structural changes at these sites. Ultrasound has been especially attractive because it emits no radiation and is remarkably mobile. It can be aimed at any blood vessel or organ and can detect with some precision modest structural changes.

Functional changes relate to the flexibility or compliance of the artery walls, which become stiffer in the presence of disease. During exercise, the arteries normally relax to accommodate more blood flow, but that function may be deficient in early disease. The heart muscle also may get stiff in early disease. When the small arteries to the kidney constrict, protein often leaks into the urine. We can detect all of these functional abnormalities in our effort to identify early disease.

Most cardiovascular disease is generalized throughout the body, not localized as in most early cancers. So the purpose of imaging methods in asymptomatic individuals is to detect the presence of disease, not to find a localized lesion in need of treatment. The question, therefore, is how sensitive and how specific these various imaging tests are and what are the side effects or unwanted consequences of using them.

SENSITIVITY AND SPECIFICITY

Sensitivity is the ability to detect the disease if it is present, and specificity is the ability to exclude the disease if it is absent. No tests are perfectly sensitive and specific, but the best tests have a high degree of both. For instance, fever is a pretty sensitive guide to the presence of a severe bacterial infection, since almost all such infections are accompanied by fever. But its specificity is low, since many people without bacterial infections may also have a fever.

The sensitivity and specificity of blood pressure measurement as a guide to cardiovascular disease is dependent on where you place the threshold for an abnormal reading. If you set it low, like over 120/80 mmHg, then the measurement becomes quite sensitive. The vast majority of individuals with cardiovascular disease have readings over 120/80 mmHg. But specificity is very low since most people with readings above 120/80 mmHg are perfectly normal. If, however, the threshold is raised to 140/90 mmHg, specificity is high and sensitivity very low. Most people with resting readings consistently above 140/90 mmHg have demonstrable early disease, but sensitivity is very low because of the large number of people with early or advanced disease who have blood pressures between 120–140/80–90 mmHg.

Heart scans, a standard test that involves radiation, detects calcium in the coronary arteries. It is highly specific since calcium exists almost only when an atherosclerotic plaque is present in the coronary artery. But it is highly insensitive because plaques that cause heart attacks may not contain calcium. Furthermore our goal is to find the early disease before the plaques develop. Disease may also exist and be equally dangerous in arteries other than the coronary arteries. Similarly, ultrasound of the carotid arteries in the neck may detect thickening of the artery wall. This thickening is usually a sign of artery disease likely to progress, but many individuals with atherosclerosis have normal carotid arteries (lack of sensitivity), and many individuals without any other evidence for disease may have thickened carotid arteries (lack of specificity).

We recognized this problem of sensitivity and specificity when we designed our Rasmussen Center for Cardiovascular Disease Prevention more than fifteen years ago. We appreciated the need for using noninvasive and preferably nonionized radiation (non-X-ray) tests to detect early disease in asymptomatic individuals. We recognized that all cardiovascular morbid events are not consequences of the same disease process. Heart attacks, or myocardial infarction, result from blockages in the large coronary arteries that run on the surface of the heart. Most strokes result from blockages or rupture of the large arteries that supply the brain. Heart failure results from an alteration in function and structure of the pumping chamber of the heart, the left ventricle. Sudden death results from an electrical defect in the signaling that keeps the heart beat synchronous, and it is almost always accompanied by structural changes in the heart. Disturbances in the circulation to the legs results from blockages in those large arteries as well as small arteries. Circulation problems to the kidney leading to kidney failure are most often due to narrowing of the small, microscopic arteries that supply the kidney. Similarly, dementia, often called Alzheimer's disease, may be a consequence of small, microscopic artery obstruction in the brain.

These sites of vascular disease cannot be detected by any one test. So we designed a series of ten noninvasive and non-X-ray tests that could be completed in one room in one hour and that allowed us to detect abnormalities of function or structure of the large arteries, the small microscopic arteries, and the left ventricle.[5] The studies include measurement of blood pressure not only at rest but also in response to a modest three-minute exercise on a treadmill. Exercise induces a rise in blood pressure that is accentuated when the blood vessels are stiff and when nitric oxide is deficient. We also measure the stiffness of small arteries and large arteries from a waveform recorded with a sensor placed on the wrist. A retinal camera is used to record a digital picture of the small arteries in the back of the eye, and an ultrasound examination of the large carotid arteries in the neck provides a measure of their thickness and detects any plaques that may have formed in the artery wall. A urine test for protein (albumin), an ultrasound examination of the heart, an electrocardiogram, and a blood test for a hormone, NT-ProBNP, that is secreted in excess when the heart is under strain complete the examination.

By giving each test a score, which we sum to get a Disease Score, we are able to assess the degree of severity of disease, not at a single site but in the entire circulatory system. The Disease Score has turned out to be both highly sensitive and highly specific in detecting the likelihood of future cardiovascular morbid events.[6] The Disease Score, therefore, tells you how far your "car" is "down the road" at your age. If your "speed" will likely get you to age one hundred before you reach the road's end, we recommend no treatment. If, however, the Disease Score suggests you are at risk for a premature morbid event, then we suggest lifestyle or drug treatment, which is always individualized.

WHAT INFLUENCES THE DISEASE SCORE?

It's not surprising that the Disease Score is influenced by factors that are known to be associated with cardiovascular morbid events. Age is the most obvious. Some of the individual test scores are adjusted for age, but even so, the Disease Score tends to rise with age because cardiovascular functional and structural changes progress with age. A healthy sixty-year-old has stiffer and thicker arteries than a healthy forty-year-old, so even with adjustment, older individuals generally have higher scores for disease than do young individuals. People with higher blood pressure have more disease than those with lower blood pressure. Women have just as much disease as men, and cholesterol levels have only a minor influence on the severity of disease. Even obesity is less a contributor than you might think. Yes, obese individuals have somewhat more disease, but many obese and overweight people are remarkably free from disease.

The story that emerges from our data is that people must be individually evaluated. They should not be treated exclusively on the basis of some measurement like weight, blood pressure, or gender. These may offer a statistical likelihood, but individualized evaluation and targeted treatment are the preferred strategy.

Remember the basketball team chosen by height alone. A short team of talented players will beat them every time.

DOES THE DISEASE SCORE CHANGE OVER TIME?

One of the remarkable advantages of using the Disease Score is that it can be repeated at intervals to determine the rate, if any, of disease progression (how fast the car is going down the highway). Rather than waiting to determine if a patient has a heart attack or stroke, we can monitor over time to see if the therapy prescribed is having a favorable effect on the rate of progression. Even more important, perhaps, we can repeat studies on individuals who may have decided not to take prescribed medications because of their concern for side effects. If disease is progressing, we find they often become more compliant.

We have now completed studies of several of the drugs we routinely prescribe for patients with high Disease Scores. When compared to placebo pills in patients who are not aware of which drug they are taking, these drugs have produced quite striking reductions in Disease Score over durations of nine months to a year.[7] These drugs have the potential to effectively "apply the brakes." The ability to monitor patients over time provides the opportunity to individualize therapy. If a patient displays progression of disease, then the current management strategy is inadequate and should be changed. If progression has stopped, then the patient should be encouraged to continue the current therapy. This knowledge empowers the patient and the caregiver.

WHAT ARE THE ARGUMENTS AGAINST EARLY DETECTION?

It is almost incomprehensible that there is a strong attitude among many medical experts that the search for early disease in asymptomatic adults is not justified. I say "incomprehensible" because the frequency of cardiovascular morbid events terminating a healthy life in previously asymptomatic adults is very high, much higher than the incidence of breast cancer and colon cancer for which early detection is championed by most of the same authorities.

Health-care authorities focus on two groups of individuals who they view as at high risk. The first are individuals who have already survived a cardiovascular morbid event—perhaps a heart attack, a stroke, or symptoms leading to stent placement in a coronary artery. These patients are in need of secondary prevention, which includes drug therapy they may not be receiving. It is indeed depressing to see how many of these individuals with well-established disease are not receiving drugs that we know can slow further disease progression. The second are patients with persistently high blood pressure or high cholesterol levels, which identify them as likely to be at high risk for a morbid event and in need of drug therapy to reduce that risk.

Concern for these groups is entirely appropriate. They are statistically at a higher risk and treatment can be justified. They can be identified without searching for the presence of early disease. Those with a prior morbid event have already demonstrated that they have advanced cardiovascular disease. There is no need to search for early disease. They need treatment to slow further progression, but their disease has probably already progressed. In the analogy of the car on the highway, the car may be already approaching the end of the road. "Applying the brakes" at this point may delay the fatal crash, but long-term survival may be limited.

Aiming therapy at elevated risk factor levels is a little more complicated. Yes, many of those with high LDL-cholesterol levels may not have early disease and therefore may be needlessly treated. I would prefer to evaluate them for early disease before initiating therapy, but I understand the reluctance of the guidelines to recommend such evaluation before initiating statin therapy, especially if the LDL levels are very high, such as 190 mg%, which greatly increases the likelihood of atherosclerotic disease. In patients reluctant to take a statin drug, demonstration of early blood vessel disease often convinces them of the need. In the hypertensive individual, especially when resting blood pressure is higher than 150/100 mmHg, the likelihood of early blood vessel disease is so high (more than 80 percent) that drug treatment without a search for early disease can be justified. In those with lower levels of hypertension, however, or those with fluctuating blood pressure levels, evaluation for early disease is essential in order to initiate individualized therapy.

The problem with the current approach, however, is not so much the unnecessary treatment of individuals mistakenly thought to be at risk, but nontreatment of those with early disease who do not exhibit any risk factors for which guidelines recommend therapy. More than half the heart attacks in the United States today occur in individuals who are not on risk-factor treatment and do not have risk-factor levels that experts believe need treatment. That is the group that is not being identified and not being treated to prevent these events. These are also the individuals whose "cars" may only be a short way "down the road" and in whom targeted therapy may slow its speed so they can reach the coveted one hundredth birthday. These are individuals in need of evaluation for early disease.

The opposition to early disease detection is also based on operational issues, not conceptual ones. Testing that involves local imaging alone often leads to unnecessary localized procedures that are expensive, traumatic, and not justified. Our screening includes no testing that should lead to inappropriate localized intervention. Sensitivity and specificity are concerns and lead to controversies about cost-effectiveness. No large-scale trials have been done to document the cost and effectiveness of efforts to detect early disease. Does it prevent morbid events and does it reduce or at least not increase health-care costs?

Such trials to document cost-effectiveness of this approach are urgently needed. The problem is that trials such as these require many participants and long follow-up. They are very expensive. Trials to document effectiveness of a drug to reduce morbidity or mortality in a population with disease may cost as much as $300 million. Even larger studies would be required in a healthy population in whom morbid events may be considerably less frequent. Who will pay for these studies?

Funding agencies must be convinced that the future of health care should be to prevent disease rather than to focus only on better and more expensive methods to treat disease. The latter approach threatens to bankrupt our health-care budget. Prevention is the only solution to these escalating costs.

The other reason why some experts criticize the attempt to identify early disease in need of treatment is their perception that the effort is unnecessary. They have convinced themselves that our current effort at detecting and controlling risk factors is the only data needed to control the epidemic of cardiovascular disease. These experts have been so brainwashed by the epidemiologic focus on risk factors that they have come to believe risk-factor control is all that is needed. Those risk factors obviously include obesity, high blood pressure, high cholesterol, and smoking. Control these factors, the current mantra goes, and we will eliminate the epidemic.

If this formulation is not correct, how did the concept gain such power? Well, there is an element of truth in the mantra. The rate of progression of atherosclerosis is influenced by all these risk factors, to an individually variable degree. Smokers, particularly, usually suffer from an accelerated process. Each of these risk factors, when studied in a large population, is associated with an excess of morbid events. The magnitude of that acceleration is highly statistically significant; that is, it is not a chance relationship. But its magnitude is rather modest. Eliminating smoking, obesity, dietary indiscretion, and elevated blood pressure would significantly reduce the frequency of cardiovascular disease in our society. It might reduce events by 20 or even 30 percent, a profound reduction in a disease now costing American society over a trillion dollars a year.

Then why is the mantra misleading? It isn't, if your ultimate goal is to reduce the excess deaths directly related to these risk factors. But if your goal is more ambitious, as is mine, the challenge is to eliminate all cardiovascular morbid events prior to age one hundred. It is to slow the trajectory of disease progression in everyone with disease, not just the modest fraction whose disease can be attributed in part to the risk factors. That means the population at risk for these events without the influence of risk-factor elevations deemed to be in need of treatment. That means the large population, perhaps half of all Americans, whose disease is quietly progressing without their knowing it.

How can this be accomplished? How can we evaluate the whole population to identify this subset? And how can we reliably slow the rate of progression, even if we can find the disease?

We shall discuss this in chapter 13.

CONFLICT OF INTEREST

Whenever an innovative diagnostic or therapeutic approach is developed, it is incumbent on the developer to seek intellectual property rights. Further development and expanded usage of these innovative approaches are dependent on an economic incentive that accompanies patent protection. I have in the course of my career obtained patents on a number of diagnostic and therapeutic approaches, some of which are still generating modest royalty revenue.

When I developed the Disease Score, which was a unique way to assess the presence and severity of early vascular disease, I sought through the University of Minnesota a patent that might encourage further development and expansion of its use. That led to the establishment of a limited liability corporation dedicated to documenting the sensitivity and specificity of the methodology and attempting to expand its usage beyond the University of Minnesota.

That process has slowly expanded. The approach is still in its infancy but now has the possibility of becoming a larger enterprise dedicated to improving preventive health care nationwide. Investors in the corporation share the goal to spread the technology worldwide.

When one promotes a product that one has developed, it is natural to challenge the integrity of the promoter. But when one has developed the product to improve well-being, its promotion can appropriately be considered an extension of the creative process. I have always believed we need to be more effective in our efforts to identify early disease. The Disease Score I developed has brought us closer to that goal. I feel I need not apologize for promoting it.

Nonetheless, a developer's support for his own innovation is always suspect. When there is a financial award for its success, suspicion should be even higher. Documentation of the sensitivity and specificity of the Disease Score, and its utility in improving preventive management, must come from others. My biases will always generate a challenge to my objectivity in evaluating the effectiveness of our approach.

CONTEMPORARY UNDERSTANDING

- Early vascular and cardiac disease can be detected by a one-hour non-invasive evaluation that need not be expensive.
- Most of the individuals found to have early disease do not present with risk factors at a level for which therapy is currently recommended.
- Targeted treatment can slow progression of this early disease.
- The earlier the abnormalities are detected, the more effective the therapy to slow their progression can be.

13

SECONDARY PREVENTION

CONVENTIONAL WISDOM

- Secondary prevention is aimed at individuals with known disease who have suffered at least one cardiovascular morbid event.
- The goal is to prevent subsequent morbid events in individuals who are at high risk because they have had a prior cardiovascular event.
- The data on effective treatment is well established in such individuals because of the wealth of clinical trials in this population.
- Everyone who has had a prior event should certainly be on treatment, if tolerated, with drugs known to be effective in preventing recurrent events.

CLASSIFICATION OF PREVENTIVE EFFORTS

Health experts have in recent years divided efforts to prevent cardiovascular disease into three categories. Primordial prevention is focused on community interventions to reduce the prevalence of elevated blood pressure, obesity, and other so-called risk factors in the community. Primary prevention is aimed at healthy individuals in an effort to reduce their personal risk by adopting certain lifestyle or even drug interventions. Secondary prevention is aimed at individuals who already have had symptoms of cardiovascular disease, such as a heart attack, stroke, or heart failure. These are individuals we know have disease. They have already consumed considerable health-care resources. The goal is to prevent recurrences.

Primordial prevention is not conceptually a responsibility of physicians or health-care providers. It is a community-based effort aimed at altering the environment, encouraging exercise, and trying to influence the availability of healthy foods in the marketplace. The cost of instituting such programs in schools and in the community is justified by the concept that a lower rate of morbid events will save more money on health care than the programs cost to carry out.

Primordial prevention is only potentially as effective as is the role of environmental factors in determining the risk of cardiovascular morbid events. If most of the individual risk is related to genomics, then environmental intervention can have only a small impact on relative risk. Here is where the future of genomic medicine has its richest potential, but the complexity of multigenetic influences on the risk of cardiovascular disease in individuals, each of whom is genetically distinct, makes the use of genomic data to determine risk very elusive. And of course intervening by altering genetic predilection is beyond the grasp of current biology. If the purpose of genetic testing is to identify individuals at risk in order to intervene with lifestyle changes or drugs, then identifying early disease in need of treatment would seem to be the more effective strategy. Genetic predilections are translated into disease only by acceleration of the biological process.

Primary prevention is a more complicated challenge. The burden falls on primary care providers. Their dedication to this effort varies immensely. Some take on the responsibility to serve their patients with comprehensive preventive efforts, but others are more concerned with dealing with symptomatic disease episodes. Preventive efforts such as mammography and colonoscopy to identify early cancer are well-established by guidelines. Primary caregivers need only order these procedures to be done. Preventive efforts for cardiovascular disease are less clear. Guidelines suggest that everyone's personal data should be entered into a calculator of ten-year risk, using either the traditional Framingham database[1] or the more recent AHA/ACC algorithm.[2] What the practitioner should do with such data is less clear.

There are many choices that practitioners can make. If the ten-year risk is high, such as 10 or even 20 percent, they could consider prescribing a drug, such as a statin or an antihypertensive agent, but these latter agents are generally used to treat specific levels of blood pressure, not risk alone. For the caregiver, this may not be a problem because a high risk on these algorithms almost always means that the blood pressure is elevated, since the blood pressure is an important contributor to the calculated risk. The practitioner may also suggest the daily use of a baby aspirin, if the patient is not already taking it. The media often trumpets the benefits of a daily aspirin to prevent heart attacks, but the most recent guidelines, while recognizing the data indicating the protective value of this drug, also point out the risk of bleeding that leads them to advising doctors to evaluate the individual's risk and benefits before prescribing the drug. How the doctor is supposed to do that remains unclear. The goal of aspirin is of course to prevent clots that may form on atherosclerotic plaques in the coronary or cerebral circulation. But the data supporting its use remain controversial, and despite the overall safety record of low-dose aspirin, bleeding does occur and can be life-threatening.

The message to primary caregivers regarding primary prevention is mostly to encourage their patients to follow the population-based approach to prevention: eat a prudent diet, exercise regularly, and keep your weight down. The higher your risk score, if you calculate it from standard demographic data algorithms, the more aggressively you should pursue this lifestyle. That's the same message that communities are delivering in their promotion of primordial prevention. That generic message should not, I emphasize, be the job of caregivers. They should be evaluating the individual and providing recommendations specific to that individual.

The widely emphasized general recommendation that the intensity of treatment should match the magnitude of the risk is a population-based concept, not one based on concern for the individual.[3] If the population, however one selects it, exhibits traits that are associated with a high risk, the recommendation is that this population deserves aggressive therapy, regardless of the likelihood that within the population are individuals at no risk. Furthermore, no therapy may be recommended for a population at low risk, even if individuals within that population have advancing disease that needs treatment. This population approach does not well serve the individual. It is aimed at balancing the benefits and risks in a population, not selecting the optimal approach for an individual.

Secondary prevention is comparatively simple. Everyone in that category has the disease of interest, and your goal is to slow its progression and prevent future morbid events. Multiple studies have been carried out in people who have suffered such events, so there is a rich database demonstrating the benefit of various interventions. Expert panels have reviewed these data and have promoted recommendations on how caregivers should treat various individuals who have had certain disease events. The guidelines are quite clear.

But what muddies the water is the question of when secondary prevention begins. There is no question that someone who has had a myocardial infarction has coronary atherosclerosis likely to result in a future heart attack. But what if he or she is asymptomatic but has calcium in the coronary arteries, a sure sign of atherosclerosis? Is that patient a candidate for secondary prevention or primary prevention? Should the guidelines for secondary prevention be followed or rather the nebulous guidelines for primary prevention? Or what if there is a cholesterol plaque visualized by ultrasound of the carotid artery in the neck? Is that evidence for disease and the need for secondary prevention, or is that still primary prevention? When in the course of a progressive disease process that advances over decades does primary prevention merge into secondary prevention? Do we need to wait for a morbid event, which is costly, may be fatal, and may leave the patient with a reduced quality of life? Or can we start secondary prevention as soon as disease can be recognized in the arteries or heart, especially if it appears to suggest an acceleration of the normal aging process? The emergence of simple, noninvasive ways to identify early disease is challenging the current definition of secondary prevention. Since the disease is age-dependent, when in the progressive course of early cardiovascular disease is it appropriate to decide the patient needs secondary prevention? When does the individual join the "club" of people who need drug therapy to protect them from future morbid events?

FAILURE OF THE HEALTH-CARE SYSTEM

The task of identifying individuals who have suffered a cardiovascular morbid event should be quite simple. The guidelines mandating that such individuals receive preventive drug therapy are clear. Then why are so many individuals who fit that description not receiving appropriate preventive therapy?[4] Is it the fault of their doctors, themselves, or the health-care system? Regardless of who is at fault, the result is a very high recurrence rate that fills our hospitals, consumes billions of dollars in medical costs that could have been prevented, shortens survival, and impairs quality of life in millions.

It is hard to know where to place the blame. Most patients do not like taking pills, so there is a natural reluctance that can influence the primary care provider not to write a prescription or the patient not to fill it. Most importantly, such preventive therapy probably must be taken for life, and there is a high attrition rate for continuing therapy when the patient feels well. One could certainly justify a national policy of free preventive therapy that could eliminate the economic incentive to discontinue effective preventive therapy.

The problem of dealing with more subtle evidence for disease, such as the evaluation process described in the last chapter, is more complex. Since these individuals have no symptoms of disease or a prior morbid event, they must be studied in order to document the artery or heart disease. Guidelines do not generally recommend such evaluation. The disease in such individuals is like an iceberg where most of the problem is under the water and invisible. The health-care system has so far discouraged looking under the water. They deny the presence and importance of this early disease at their own peril. The health-care system may be viewed as the *Titanic* heading for an unrecognized disaster.

CONTEMPORARY UNDERSTANDING

- The traditional distinction between primary and secondary prevention is no longer viable.
- Preventive therapy should be aimed not so much at preventing morbid events but at slowing disease progression.
- Cardiovascular disease progresses with age in everyone. When its rate of progression portends a premature morbid event, treatment to slow progression should be administered.
- Treatment to slow progression should be so effective in decreasing health-care costs that a national policy of free medication is justified.

14

A COMMUNITY APPROACH

CONVENTIONAL WISDOM

- Health care in the community is managed by primary care providers (PCPs).
- Specialists are utilized only to deal with overt organ system disease.
- Preventive efforts are overseen by PCPs, who enforce the community-wide effort to prevent and/or neutralize risk factors.
- Reducing hospitalizations and death from cardiovascular disease by even 10 percent is a worthwhile community goal and could produce a substantial reduction in health-care costs.

RATIONALE FOR THE STRATEGY

The aim to eliminate symptomatic cardiovascular disease (morbid events) prior to age one hundred involves detection and effective management of asymptomatic early disease likely to progress. Well over 50 percent of heart attacks and strokes occur in patients who have had no prior warning signs that they have underlying and progressive disease of their arteries or heart. But they do. Heart attacks and strokes, which result from obstruction or rupture of arteries, do not occur in normal arteries. Except in the unusual instances where the clot arrives in the artery from another site where disease is known to exist, the culprit artery is always chronically involved with a process called atherosclerosis. It is finding that atherosclerosis that is one of the vital goals of the detection process.

Diseases of the heart, like heart failure, do not develop suddenly in a previously normal heart. Structural changes in the heart muscle long precede the development of the symptomatic condition called heart failure. If the heart's pumping capacity becomes impaired, that impairment can be detected long before symptoms develop. So assessing the structure and function of the heart, which can now be done quite simply with ultrasound techniques, is a valuable way to identify disease before it becomes symptomatic.

But even if we can justify the benefit of detecting the early asymptomatic disease, and even if there is strong evidence that treatment aimed at slowing its progression can prevent morbid events, how would it be possible to evaluate and treat an entire population? How can we logistically accomplish such a community-wide screening, and how can we bear the cost? Isn't this just an approach that might apply to a small subset of the affluent population? Are we advocating an approach for the top 1 percent or for everyone?

THE PLAN

In reviewing our test data from individuals evaluated in our Rasmussen Center for Cardiovascular Disease Prevention, we made an important observation. Whereas most of the testing involves complex instrumentation and technical expertise, four of our ten tests are quite simple to perform and require little training to do so. These four tests provide a remarkably comprehensive assessment of the health of the arteries that are the direct cause of most cardiovascular morbid events. When we examined the scores on these four tests in more than 2,000 individuals we had evaluated in Minneapolis, we found that a score of 3 or more on these four tests correctly identified 90 percent of the individuals whose total score was at least 6 and who were in need of drug therapy. We then reviewed the findings in more than 2,000 individuals evaluated in a program we had established in Sarasota, Florida. In this population, which was somewhat older, the four tests were accurate in identifying progressive disease in 91 percent of the population.

The four-test screening can't replace the ten-test program because the full evaluation is necessary to provide a comprehensive assessment of the cardiovascular system in order to devise a treatment plan. Nonetheless the screening is 90 percent reliable in identifying individuals with enough early disease to require treatment. Thus, if you are willing to be 90 percent correct (it's a lot better than a flip of the coin, but it's not perfect), then these four tests can be utilized to exclude individuals who need not be concerned about their cardiovascular health and need not take preventive therapy. They can be encouraged to return at three- to five-year intervals for rescreening.

Fortunately these four rather simple tests can be set up in any clinic where PCPs see patients, and the tests can be easily performed by clinic staff without much special training. We have established this testing in a clinic in suburban Minneapolis, and it is working very well. Other sites are in the planning stage.

Who should we screen with this four-test approach? We started out thinking screening was appropriate for all adults. But there are some identifiable groups in whom the incidence of disease is so low that screening them is probably not cost-effective. We have therefore excluded from the screening individuals who are thin, have no family history of cardiovascular disease, have no traits or diseases that place them at higher risk, and have blood pressure and cholesterol levels on the low side of normal. We may miss some early disease in these individuals but they may always come back for future evaluation.

What percentage of healthy, asymptomatic, self-referred adults going through the four tests have scores high enough to place them at risk and to mandate the full ten-test evaluation, which means referral to a central site with appropriate instrumentation and staff? In Minnesota it is 36 percent and in Sarasota 32 percent. This experience does not include our planned exclusion of very low-risk individuals, which we expect will increase the rate of abnormal four-test scores to about 60 percent. We are anxious to test other population groups to begin to get a handle on the community incidence of early cardiovascular disease. We also need to continuously remind ourselves that about half of American adults will die or be disabled by cardiovascular disease, so early cardiovascular disease, if it is indeed a harbinger of future morbid events, should be present in more than half the population.

BLOOD PRESSURE

Blood pressure measurement is a simple procedure that is part of our four-test screening. It is a key marker for cardiovascular disease, not only because high blood pressure is a well-known risk factor for vascular and heart disease, but also because disease in the arteries themselves will tend to raise blood pressure. When small arteries stiffen or thicken, as they do in atherosclerosis, the blood flowing through these small tubes encounters resistance to flow that raises the pressure of blood pumped by the heart. For the amount of blood pumped by the heart to remain constant in order to nourish the tissues, a higher resistance to flow demands the heart to generate a higher pressure.

Blood pressure is measured in every health-care provider's office. Such measurements are also available in drug stores, health clubs, and fire houses. Today many people buy their own apparatus at a neighborhood drug store and check their own pressure at home. Hopefully the conditions for measurement of a resting, sitting blood pressure are more standardized in our clinics than those confronted in the drug store or health club, but the technique is not very different. One difference is our criterion for normal. Less than 130/85 mmHg gets a normal rating in our center, or a score of zero. Over 140/90 mmHg gets an abnormal score, or +2. In between, a condition that might be labeled as pre-hypertension in some clinics, the score is borderline, or +1.

The critical second test in our clinic assessment is the blood pressure during exercise. The devotion of our health-care system to resting blood pressure and its use to drive medical management of hypertension disregards the well-known dramatic influence of exercise on blood pressure. Since most of us are not sedentary throughout the day, the blood pressure during daily activity, including exercise, may be a more important guide to the health of our arteries and heart. We use a treadmill to standardize a three-minute exercise test, setting the treadmill at a work load of 5 METS, a standardization that combines treadmill speed and slope. This 5 MET workload is a modest walking pace that everyone should be capable of performing with little effort. We measure the blood pressure at the end of the three minutes to determine how much it has changed. We have normal, borderline, and abnormal ranges for the blood pressure change.

ARTERY STIFFNESS

The other screening tests take advantage of a device we developed some twenty years ago to calculate the stiffness separately of the large arteries and the small arteries.[1] It is a device placed around the wrist to analyze the pulse wave in the radial artery on the thumb side of the wrist. The device, a transducer, is placed over the pulse and transmits the waveform to a screen where it can be visualized. A computer program analyzes the waveform, from which it can calculate separately a value for small artery elasticity or stiffness and large artery elasticity or stiffness. The stiffer the arteries, the greater the severity of the disease. Our numbers for normal (score 0), borderline (score +1), and abnormal (score +2) differ depending on the age and gender of the individual being tested.

Performing these four tests usually takes less than fifteen minutes. If the total score of the four tests is 2 or less, we consider the testing normal and do not refer the patient for more extensive testing. We do, however, encourage them to come back at three- to five-year intervals for retesting. Scores of 3 or greater place the patient at high risk for progressive disease, which justifies their referral to the evaluation center for more comprehensive assessment.

One advantage of these four screening tests is that they respond very well to treatment. The drug therapy that we generally prescribe for patients with progressive disease includes drugs that lower both resting blood pressure and the rise in blood pressure with exercise as well as improve the elasticity or stiffness of the small arteries. So these tests not only identify individuals with a greater likelihood of early disease, but they can also be utilized to document a therapeutic response.

Why do we separately assess large artery and small artery stiffness? The large arteries, which are arteries you can feel and see, are the usual site of obstructions that cause heart attacks and strokes. They stiffen because of thickening of their walls, a structural change that generally accompanies atherosclerosis. Those structural changes are not easily reversible. On the other hand, the small, microscopic arteries stiffen because of both functional and structural abnormalities. The early stiffening occurs because of narrowing of the artery without structural change, probably a consequence of endothelial dysfunction or nitric oxide deficiency. That constriction is reversible with treatment, and the sooner the intervention, the more effective the treatment will be in reversing the stiffening and restoring the small arteries to normal.[2]

THE COMMUNITY STRATEGY

The effort to gain access to the entire community and provide evaluation and management recommendations for all at-risk individuals is a long-term project, but it can start immediately. The plan involves access to primary care providers, eventually all in a given community. A four-test screening in all patients under the physician's care is certainly achievable and would add only fifteen to twenty minutes to a regular visit. Those testing positive would be referred for full evaluation, a process that takes over an hour at a central site where the full screening program can be carried out. Over the course of a year, a single technologist can reasonably provide a full evaluation of about 1,400 patients. In a community of 100,000 adults, perhaps 40,000 would be at-risk and in need of full evaluation. Six technologists working at perhaps three central sites would be able to evaluate the entire at-risk adult population in about five years, thus making it possible to re-evaluate at appropriate intervals to track progression of disease.

A key to the success of such a program is the enthusiastic support of the primary care community. Recommendations for individualized therapy of patients who test positive are provided to the primary care provider with the assumption that they will act on the recommendations. Failure to prescribe the recommended therapy or failure to encourage compliance with the recommendations would threaten the proposed benefits of the program.

These estimates of the potential for such a community program are at best very preliminary attempts to quantify the practicality of the program. Its costs, and particularly its effectiveness, need to be established. But this proposal is presented in the hope that it will spawn a more critical assessment of a plan that, for the first time, provides a reasonable and testable approach to a community-wide slowing of disease progression and a profound reduction of cardiovascular disease morbidity.

CONTEMPORARY UNDERSTANDING

- Modern health care will require primary care providers to work in collaboration with other health-care experts to provide optimal health care.
- Cardiovascular disease prevention requires more than environmentally based risk-factor intervention. Detection of early disease and appropriate medical management to prevent its progression require cardiovascular disease assessment and the adoption of individually directed management strategies.
- The goal of eliminating cardiovascular morbid events before the age of one hundred is a rigorous challenge, but with appropriate organization and support, it is potentially achievable.

15

A FUTURE FREE OF SYMPTOMATIC CARDIOVASCULAR DISEASE

CONVENTIONAL WISDOM

- Cardiovascular disease is inevitable if you live long enough.
- If we could delay cardiovascular disease enough, it would result in an aged, demented population that would be a burden to society.
- Treatment has improved so much that cardiovascular disease morbidity can be effectively managed after it occurs.
- You have to die from something.

CAN CARDIOVASCULAR MORBID EVENTS BE ELIMINATED?

We have become so accustomed to heart attacks and strokes in older people that we have come to accept them as a normal consequence of aging. Perhaps that explains why people are so much more afraid of cancer than of cardiovascular disease. Perhaps that explains why the contributions to the American Cancer Society are so much greater than those to the American Heart Association. Heart disease is no big deal, but the "C" word . . . we don't even want to say "cancer" for fear it might strike us.

Since the vast majority of cardiovascular disease is now preventable—as opposed to cancer—it's possible to envision a society free of cardio-

vascular disease. But we can't begin in countries with emerging econo-
mies where health care is not well organized nor widely available. Rather,
we should start in the metropolitan areas of the United States where an
appropriate infrastructure is in place.

Aging of the blood vessels and heart is inevitable. It has long been
accepted that if people live long enough, they will have a cardiovascular
morbid event and die from some form of cardiovascular disease. After all,
you must die from something. So you can't eliminate cardiovascular
disease morbidity and mortality, but you can delay it.

How long should we propose delaying it? When I was in my childhood, a sixty-five-year-old seemed aged. That's when Medicare clicks in
and people are supposed to retire. Since we have always wanted them to
enjoy retirement, we'd like to extend their disease-free life for some
years, perhaps fifteen, to age eighty. But people are now healthier and
living longer, perhaps in part due to our successful efforts at managing
chronic disease. And a morbid event delayed from sixty to eighty will still
cost the health-care system the same amount of money. So morbidity can
be delayed, but costs ultimately stay the same. No one is willing to ration
health care after the age of eighty. What about ninety? Can we legislate
that health care stops at ninety? Highly unlikely, since many of our lead-
ers are approaching or have surpassed that age. So how about one hundred? A century of life seems adequate for the government to limit treatment and cost. Individuals would still be free to seek their own health
care, but Medicare would say, "Enough; you're on your own!" It would
be the secret to truly "preventing morbid events." It would avoid the cost
of morbid events, which is a critical factor in our dedication to prevention. And its aim would be to prevent cardiovascular illness until age one
hundred, a goal that most of us would accept, at least until we approach
that age.

A COMMUNITY FREE FROM PREMATURE
CARDIOVASCULAR DISEASE

What would that community look like? All people with advancing early
disease who are at risk for cardiovascular disease morbidity and mortality
would be on a regimen (likely including drugs) that would dramatically
slow progression of their underlying disease. This therapy would delay

any morbid events with a goal of event-free life to one hundred years. What would happen then? The individual would no longer be provided with government-supported care. Heart attacks and strokes would generally be cared-for at home and without efforts to prolong life. The burgeoning cost of cardiovascular care would be shifted from the Medicare years to the post-insurance years.

What would the dramatic expansion of elderly residents look like? Aging of the muscle, bones, and joints will likely continue unabated, so mobility assistance will be widespread. Dementia may surprisingly not be as big a problem as feared, since much of the dementia that currently afflicts the elderly is a consequence of small artery disease whose progression should be slowed by the treatment. Admittedly, this concept is yet to be adequately tested. Cancer will likely become the major cause of death, at least until we develop better and nondestructive tools to prevent it.

HOW CAN WE TREAT THE WHOLE COMMUNITY?

One strategy promulgated by population scientists and discussed in a prior chapter is the polypill, which would be made available "over the counter." This approach accepts the concept that disease progression can be effectively slowed. Rather than expending the effort to identify individuals at risk and tailor therapy for individuals, the goal would be to administer a cocktail of medications, albeit perhaps in inadequate doses, to every adult in the community. This cocktail would be made up of a variety of drugs that have been demonstrated to reduce the risk of heart attacks, strokes, and other morbid events. The exact components of this pill, if all components can indeed by formulated into a single pill, are not currently known but could hopefully be developed. We can all envision impediments to this approach, including the unwillingness of everyone in the population to take such a daily medication. We would also be advocating therapy for half the population who are not at risk for such a morbid event, and we would be providing "one size fits all" therapy for an entire population even though it may be effective for only a subset. Our view is that individuals with a low score on the four-test screening should be deemed as not in need of the polypill.

The more rational approach I envision is based on the descriptions in previous chapters. Early detection of disease in need of treatment is possible and practical. The treatment plan can be tailored to the individual's abnormalities. The health-care system should be adequate to track the patient, which would certainly not be so in a polypill plan without involvement of the health-care system. The polypill may be a rational approach in emerging countries, but not in metropolitan areas of the United States.

HOW CAN WE AFFORD IT?

Cost becomes an important issue. We already spend so much on health care, you may say, how can we afford to increase it by widespread screening and treatment?

Think about it. The reason health-care costs have escalated so much is that we are doing so much more. Hospitals are teeming with patients undergoing expensive procedures and being treated with expensive devices. In my early medical career, hospitals were mainly places where patients could be observed while recuperating from their illnesses. Now they are cauldrons of activity.

Management of heart attacks and strokes is a case in point. A myocardial infarction was in the past a serious illness in which the treatment was bed rest (four to six weeks in the hospital) and close observation for complications. Now it involves a time-sensitive transport to the catheterization laboratory, where the clot in the coronary artery is identified and treated with a stent to open the artery. Expensive but life-saving!

Now strokes are being given the same priority. Instead of bed rest and rehabilitation, we now try to quickly remove the clot from an artery to the brain. This again is an example of very expensive emergency management with the benefit of an improved quality of life.

These high costs of health care result from our dedication to late-stage disease management. The teams and institutions that perform these miracle procedures are rightfully proud of their accomplishments. They have brought health care into the twenty-first century. We would never want to turn the clock back. Indeed, we must find ways to make these life-saving advances available to a much wider constituency than the affluent societies who now benefit.

But the twenty-first century must focus on preventing these expensive and life-shortening diseases. If we delay the cardiovascular morbid events to the age of one hundred, and then ration health-care expenses after the age of one hundred, we have essentially eliminated most of the escalating health-care costs that threaten our national budgets. The cost of extensive evaluation for early disease and the cost of years of medical treatment with inexpensive drugs pale beside the cost-saving of eliminating these expensive late-stage diseases.

IS DOING NOTHING AN OPTION?

Many experts claim we are doing fine as we are and should continue to advocate for diet and exercise. Their goals are limited. A modest delay in disease events is the best they can hope for, and cardiovascular health-care costs will continue to escalate. Medicare will still be responsible for all the events. They view the effort at eliminating these diseases as un-achievable and are far more committed to improved efficiency of care and developing better procedures and devices.

But there are more sinister forces at work. Health care is a monstrous-ly successful enterprise. Doctors are well-rewarded for their herculean efforts to treat these diseases. Hospitals profit from the beds occupied, facilities utilized, and procedures done. Pharmaceutical and instrument companies continue their rapid pace of developing ever-more-effective management strategies that fuel their bottom line. Insurance companies merely increase their premiums as needed to cover the cost of the bills of those insured. Everyone benefits but the population, who continue to face the risk of these life-altering morbid events, most of which would be preventable.

The only way to bring down the cost of our skewed effort is to replace our current health-care system with a single-payer system in which reduc-ing the cost—by preventing preventable disease—would become a prior-ity. That and, of course, a recognition that the government's responsibil-ity for your health care ceases at one hundred years of age.

JOINING THE "CLUB" AND SLOWING THE CAR

I have alluded in previous chapters to two analogies: joining the "club" of individuals in need of therapy to slow cardiovascular disease progression and "slowing the speed of the car" that is racing down the highway of life. These are the two essential components of our effort to prolong cardiovascular disease–free life to one hundred years.

Both components of this strategy are necessary to accomplish our goal. Those in need of treatment, the members of the "club," need to be identified. I have tried to emphasize that the health-care system's current strategy to identify these "club" members is woefully inadequate. Their strategy is to use risk factors to select members of the "club." As detailed in earlier chapters, only a minority of "club" members have risk-factor levels that would have identified them as in need of treatment. I offer a revised strategy, which we have developed and are currently testing, as an alternative. Other approaches are possible and should be tested. It is essential that we develop a way to optimally find these individuals with unrecognized disease likely to progress.

"Slowing the car" is another prerequisite to success in our endeavor. I am enthusiastic about the currently available and inexpensive drugs. With proper usage in appropriate patients, these agents can be remarkably effective in inhibiting disease progression—"slowing the car." But we have only scratched the surface of potential agents to interfere with disease progression. Better understanding of mechanisms and innovative approaches to pharmacology are likely to greatly increase our reservoir of agents that can be selectively employed to slow disease progression.

A revolution in the health-care industry is the other prerequisite for finding "club" members and "slowing the car." Recognition that slowing disease progression is the responsibility of the health-care provider would level the playing field, which is now dominated by specialists with their advanced therapeutic strategies. The system must be revised to reward excellence in preventing disease as well as excellence in treating its advanced forms. Preserving health should be a goal of every primary care provider, and the health-care system needs to develop a reward system that honors that endeavor.

IS AGE ONE HUNDRED FOR EVERYONE ACHIEVABLE?

The goal to delay cardiovascular disease morbidity and mortality to at least age one hundred is clearly not achievable in the short term. Even with appropriate use of our current pharmacologic agents, we are unlikely to achieve that level of success, even if all individuals with early disease could be identified and treated. If we were limited to our current array of therapies, the only hope of approaching that goal would be very early detection by identifying individuals with the cardiovascular disease markers at a young enough age to provide a lifelong slowing of progression.

The hidden secret to longevity for all is what has not yet been discovered. Most of the current research emphasis in cardiovascular disease has been the development of methods to replace the aging cardiovascular system with new cells, new organs, or devices. This approach accepts and even delights in the occurrence of serious cardiovascular disease events that mandate management. The current health-care reimbursement system encourages such efforts. These procedures and devices are reimbursed handsomely by our health-care insurance system. Everyone benefits, including the sick patients. But if we provide incentives for the development of drugs to interfere with aging and the disease process in the arteries and heart, it is likely that we will find exciting new compounds that will successfully halt the process.

Despite our success in utilizing already-marketed drugs to slow cardiovascular disease progression, we really do not understand how they work. Some may claim it is blood pressure reduction, but different drugs that lower blood pressure comparably have quite different effectiveness on disease progression.[1] Different drugs that lower cholesterol have quite variable effects on disease progression.[2] Effect on morbid events of these interventions is due to an effect on the arteries or the heart, not on the blood pressure or cholesterol. We need to better understand these processes to develop more targeted therapies. Disease progression can be better understood than it is now. The pharmacologic effects of drugs used to slow progression are incompletely understood. We need to challenge our basic and clinical scientists to gain further insight into the mechanisms of disease progression in order to identify safe and effective agents to slow the process. The rewards for research have been skewed in a different direction. It is time to reorient our cardiovascular research establishment to an emphasis on slowing disease progression.

We must encourage the development of effective drugs. Scientists are remarkably creative and successful when they are properly motivated. Keeping people healthy should be the goal of twenty-first-century medicine. It's an uncomfortable thought for specialists who earn their living taking care of very sick people and for entrepreneurs who have fostered the development of procedures and devices to keep people alive. But change and modernization have always driven our technological advances. We must make peace with the future and accelerate its arrival.

CONTEMPORARY UNDERSTANDING

- Cardiovascular disease is inevitable if you live long enough, but one hundred years is long enough.
- By slowing the progression of cardiovascular disease, many of the vascular ailments that affect the elderly, such as dementia, may be less debilitating than we think and the extended life may be quite rewarding.
- Our success in treating morbid events should not diminish our dedication to preventing them, a much better way to preserve health.
- The potential cost-saving of preventing cardiovascular morbid events until age one hundred far outweighs the cost of the screening and management required to accomplish it.

EPILOGUE

We have now explored a myriad of factors and mechanisms that may contribute to progression of cardiovascular disease and to the morbidity and mortality I am convinced can be prevented. I have challenged a number of messages promulgated by health authorities that insist it is your lifestyle that causes cardiovascular disease. It is not that these messages are wrong, but I think they are misleading. They have advised individuals that diet and exercise can prevent cardiovascular disease, and this message has dominated clinical behavior. Rather than encouraging individuals to understand their personal risk and intervene if necessary with drugs to slow progression, the public has been encouraged to think that drugs are a crutch for the weak, a strategy that accepts one's failure at personal behavior correction.

My advice is based on an understanding of biology, but my recommendations are largely intuitive. Our knowledge is incomplete. Nonetheless, we must act in the present, protecting ourselves as best we can based on the knowledge and intuition available to us. We must answer the question, "What can any individual do to protect himself or herself from premature cardiovascular morbid events?" That concept of "premature" may today be placed at before eighty years old, in the next ten years at before ninety, and eventually before one hundred years of age.

A PERSONAL STRATEGY

The first thing to understand is that there is no strategy appropriate for everyone. Health as well as disease is personal. Preferences for food, exercise, and mental stimulation are highly individual. Perceptions of quality of life are unique. So no advice is appropriate for everyone.

Simple principles, such as don't get fat, maintain some form of regular physical exercise, don't smoke, and drink alcohol in moderation, are standard admonitions. They are not guarantees of good health, but they probably reduce the slope of disease progression. If these activities also increase quality of life, they can be recommended with enthusiasm. Far more aggressive attempts to control diet and alter lifestyle may have a greater impact on slowing the progression of disease, but such efforts usually have an adverse effect on the joy of life. It is hard to support them when we know that pharmacologic therapy can have a remarkably favorable effect.

About age thirty-five or forty, even earlier in those with a strong family history, individuals should begin to consider their long-term cardiovascular health. Since cardiovascular disease is the most likely illness to interfere with your health and survival, disregarding your risk is a mistake.

The first step is to explore in depth your family history, if indeed it is available. Have mothers, fathers, grandparents, great-grandparents, siblings, aunts, and uncles suffered from cardiovascular diseases, such as heart attacks, strokes, heart failure, hypertension, and diabetes? This is important information and may need to be recovered from distant relatives. It is worth the effort since the tendency for cardiovascular disease is clearly inherited. A strong family history does not doom you to disease, nor is the absence of a family history a guarantee of cardiovascular health. But statistical likelihoods may be helpful in mobilizing you to action when appropriate.

The Internet these days provides you with access to genomic DNA facilities that promote analyzing your body fluids for a "personalized" approach to identify your risk. It is true that by mapping your genome, they can match you to their large databases that can calculate a percent likelihood of different future disease possibilities. But these analyses are not "personalized." In the absence of the rare conditions when a single gene fragment can be identified as the cause of a disease, these analyses can only provide statistical likelihoods. Until we can identify specific gene fragments as causative of specific medical diseases, genomic analysis will be no better than any other statistical analysis of large databases. Cardiovascular disease is in your arteries and heart, perhaps emanating from a DNA fragment or fragment combinations that we are far from being able to identify.

Once you know your family history, you can decide whether you should be very concerned, slightly concerned, or not at all concerned. Unless you come from a family that has all lived into their hundreds without cardiovascular disease, prudence should encourage you to be evaluated. Unfortunately, routine visits to your primary care provider are generally not very helpful. Your blood pressure will be checked (you can certainly do that yourself), and your cholesterol level can be measured. The doctor may do an electrocardiogram (very insensitive in detecting early disease) and might even do a stress test (unjustified in the absence of symptoms). You are likely to receive reassurance that all is well, but artery disease may still be progressing. These routine tests are not very useful in detecting early disease that may need treatment.

You and your doctor should, however, have the information needed to enter your personal data into formulae available online that will calculate your risk. These calculations are recommended by guidelines, but all doctors do not utilize them. They provide what is usually called a "ten-year risk," which means they have stacked your measurements up with a large database of similar information in thousands of other people who have been followed for at least ten years to identify heart attacks, strokes, and other major cardiovascular events. This calculation provides you a population risk, not really a personal one. If it is greater than 10 percent, or even 7.5 percent, guidelines recommend that you consider doing something about it.

I am suggesting that you do more to personalize the information. You may be referred for a cardiac scan to search for calcium in your coronary arteries. The magnitude of the calcium content does indeed provide a guide to the likelihood of a heart attack, but it is a late manifestation of disease and is rarely positive in individuals in their forties and early fifties, even if they have early artery wall disease. At that age, it is far better to search for earlier markers for disease that may progress. Treatment initiated before calcium invades the artery wall plaques is more effective than after.

I have advocated for a simple cardiovascular screening that takes about fifteen minutes. A growing number of clinics and even mobile testing laboratories are offering screening these days. Most charge out-of-pocket for this testing because it is not covered by insurance. The value of these facilities varies, but most use methods that are not very useful in detecting early disease and often do not maintain quality control in the methodology that is essential to valid results. Doctors usually have no idea what to do with the results. Our approach is two-tiered: a simple four-test screening to identify those who are unlikely to be in the "club" requiring treatment and more extensive evaluation of those at risk. The latter leads to a comprehensive medical report to the patient and the provider with specific recommendations for management. Insurance usually covers the cost.

Everyone should be aware of their risk. Blood pressure and cholesterol may influence it, and the algorithms developed by Framingham and the heart associations are very useful. Detecting early disease is even better. But regardless of how we get there, the fundamental issue is to identify the members of the "club" and get them treated to slow progression of disease.

I have not dealt in detail with the useful drugs because they are prescribed by doctors and are not available over the counter. They also may change as we gain new insights into what drives progression of disease and as new agents become available. Nonetheless, you should be made aware of the most commonly used effective drugs.

Blood-pressure-lowering drugs in general exert a favorable effect on the artery wall. It is this effect we seek when we prescribe them, especially to patients whose blood pressure is not elevated. The most effective agents inhibit the hormonal system that activates angiotensin, a potent artery constrictor and adverse artery growth stimulator. Drugs called calcium antagonists also exert a favorable effect on the arteries. That is why we often prescribe angiotensin-converting enzyme inhibitors or angiotensin receptor antagonists and amlodipine to our patients with early disease in the artery wall. These drugs are now available in single-pill combinations. Although there are differences among the individual members of these drug classes, they are probably all effective in adequate doses.

Statins are powerful agents in inhibiting the progression of atherosclerosis. Evidence for atherosclerosis leads to a prescription of one of the statin drugs, usually in a substantial dose after initiating therapy in a smaller dose. Intolerance occurs but surprisingly uncommonly. Everyone in the "club" should probably try to take a statin. The goal of this therapy is to protect the artery, not necessarily to lower the cholesterol to a target level.

These drugs are generally introduced for lifelong therapy. Once the disease is found to be accelerating, it is likely to progress in the absence of drug treatment. Lifestyle adjustments are probably unlikely to be adequate to replace drug therapy. Other drugs may also be prescribed on an individual basis. As we learn more about the disease and try new approaches, we hope to lead the way into exploration of the mechanistic and therapeutic unknown.

An often unstated benefit of our approach is to the individual whose testing shows no early disease. They can appropriately feel reassured, not permanently but certainly until the next screening, which should be soon enough to track new onset of measurable disease. Depending on age, an interval of three to five years makes sense.

Is all this effort justified? Is slowing the progression of cardiovascular disease such a big deal? I think it is. Most of us will die because of it. Both my parents died too young from cardiovascular disease. I am convinced that proper diagnosis and treatment can be effective in substantial life prolongation. If you love life, as I do, that should be reason enough to persevere.

So here is my advice. While the steak is on the grill this evening, raise a glass of red wine, swallow your statin and ACE inhibitor, grab a handful of nuts, and toast a future without cardiovascular disease.

NOTES

INTRODUCTION

1. Sanders T. Frank, "Aural Sign of Coronary Artery Disease," *New England Journal of Medicine* 289, no. 6 (1973): 327–28.

2. A. S. Go et al., "Heart Disease and Stroke Statistics—2013 Update: A Report from the American Heart Association," *Circulation* 127, no. 1 (2013): e6–e245.

3. *Diagnostic and Statistical Manual of Mental Disorders (DSM-5)* (Washington, DC: American Psychiatric Association, 2013).

1. WHAT CAUSES HEART ATTACKS, STROKES, AND OTHER CARDIOVASCULAR ILLNESSES?

1. W. A. Newman Dorland, *Dorland's Medical Dictionary* (Philadelphia: Elsevier/Saunders, 2011).

2. M. F. O'Rourke, *Arterial Function in Health and Disease* (London: Churchill Livingston, 1982).

3. Michael E. Safar and Gerard M. London, "Arterial and Venous Compliance in Sustained Essential Hypertension," *Hypertension* 10, no. 2 (1987): 133–39.

4. D. A. Duprez et al., "Determinants of Radial Artery Pulse Wave Analysis in Asymptomatic Individuals," *American Journal of Hypertension* 17, no. 8 (2004): 647–53.

5. A. J. Linzbach, "Heart Failure from the Point of View of Quantitative Anatomy," *American Journal of Cardiology* 5 (1960): 370–82.

6. D. M. Lloyd-Jones et al., "Prediction of Lifetime Risk for Cardiovascular Disease by Risk Factor Burden at 50 Years of Age," *Circulation* 113 (2006): 791–98.

7. R. B. D'Agostino Sr., R. S. Vasan, M. J. Pencina, P. A. Wolf, M. Cobain, and J. M. Massaro, "General Cardiovascular Risk Profile for Use in Primary Care: The Framingham Heart Study," *Circulation* 117, no. 6 (2008): 743–53.

8. D. Ettehad et al., "Blood Pressure Lowering for Prevention of Cardiovascular Disease and Death: A Systematic Review and Meta-analysis," *Lancet* 387, no. 10022 (2016): 957–67.

2. MYOCARDIAL INFARCTION OR HEART ATTACK

1. GISSI (Gruppo Italiano per lo Studio Della Streptochinasi Nell'Infarto Miocardico), "Effectiveness of Intravenous Thrombolytic Treatment in Acute Myocardial Infarction," *Lancet* 1, no. 8478 (1986): 397–402.

2. E. M. Antman et al., "ACC/AHA Guidelines for the Management of Patients with ST-Elevation Myocardial Infarction; A Report of the American College of Cardiology/American Heart Association Task Force on Practice Guidelines (Committee to Revise the 1999 Guidelines for the Management of Patients with Acute Myocradial Infarction)," *Journal of the American College of Cardiology* 44, no. 3 (2004): E1–E211.

3. J. S. Alpert, K. Thygesen, E. Antman, and J. P. Bassand, "Myocardial Infarction Redefined—A Consensus Document of the Joint European Society of Cardiology/American College of Cardiology Committee for the Redefinition of Myocardial Infarction," *Journal of the American College of Cardiology* 36, no. 3 (2000): 959–69.

4. C. K. Friedberg, *Diseases of the Heart*, 2nd ed. (Philadephia: W. B. Saunders Company, 1956).

5. H. M. Krumholz et al., "Reduction in Acute Myocardial Infarction Mortality in the United States: Risk-Standardized Mortality Rates from 1995–2006," *Journal of the American Medical Association* 302, no. 7 (2009): 767–73.

6. A. M. Gerdes et al., "Structural Remodeling of Cardiac Myocytes in Patients with Ischemic Cardiomyopathy," *Circulation* 86, no. 2 (1992): 426–30.

7. W. F. Enos, R. H. Homes, and J. Beyer, "Coronary Disease among United States Soldiers Killed in Action in Korea; Preliminary Report," *Journal of the American Medical Association* 152, no. 12 (1953): 1090–93.

8. M. Naghavi et al., "From Vulnerable Plaque to Vulnerable Patient: A Call for New Definitions and Risk Assessment Strategies: Part I." *Circulation* 108, no. 14 (2003): 1664–72.

9. C. Templin et al., "Clinical Features and Outcomes of Takotsubo (Stress) Cardiomyopathy," *New England Journal of Medicine* 373 (2015): 929–38.

10. C. N. Bairey Merz, "Women and Ischemic Heart Disease Paradox and Pathophysiology," *JACC Cardiovascular Imaging* 4, no. 1 (2011): 74–77.

3. BLOOD PRESSURE

1. W. D. Hall, "Stephen Hales: Theologian, Botanist, Physiologist, Discoverer of Hemodynamics," *Clinical Cardiology* 10, no. 8 (1987): 487–89.

2. J. Booth, "A Short History of Blood Pressure Measurement," *Proceedings of the Royal Society of Medicine* 70, no. 11 (1977): 793–99.

3. VA Coop Study, "Effects of Treatment on Morbidity in Hypertension. II. Results in Patients with Diastolic Blood Pressure Averaging 90 through 114 mm Hg," *Journal of the American Medical Association* 213, no. 7 (1970): 1143–52.

4. S. S. Franklin, "Ageing and Hypertension: The Assessment of Blood Pressure Indices in Predicting Coronary Heart Disease," *Journal of Hypertension Supplement* 17, no. 5 (1999): S29–36.

5. "Prevention of Stroke by Antihypertensive Drug Treatment in Older Persons with Isolated Systolic Hypertension: Final Results of the Systolic Hypertension in Elderly Program (SHEP), SHEP Cooperative Research Group," *Journal of the American Medical Association* 265, no. 24 (1991): 3255–64.

6. S. Lewington, R. Clarke, N. Qizilbash, R. Peto, and R. Collins, and Prospective Studies Collaboration, "Age-Specific Relevance of Usual Blood Pressure to Vascular Mortality: A Meta-analysis of Individual Data for One Million Adults in 61 Prospective Studies," *Lancet* 360, no. 9349 (2002): 1903–13.

7. R. S. Vasan et al., "Impact of High-Normal Blood Pressure on the Risk of Cardiovascular Disease," *New England Journal of Medicine* 345, no. 18 (2001): 1291–97.

8. A. V. Chobanian et al., "The Seventh Report of the Joint National Committee on Prevention, Detection, Evaluation and Treatment of High Blood Pressure: The JNC 7 report," *Journal of the American Medical Association* 289, no. 19 (2003): 2560–72.

9. L. K. Altman, "Drug Used in Emergencies Despite Warnings," *New York Times*, October 23, 1996.

10. K. Swedberg et al., "Treatment of Anemia with Darbepoetin Alfa in Systolic Heart Failure," *New England Journal of Medicine* 368 (2013): 1210–19.

11. L. Hansson et al., "Effects of Intensive Blood-Pressure Lowering and Low-Dose Aspirin in Patients with Hypertension: Principal Results of the Hypertension Optimal Treatment (HOT) Randomised Trial, HOT Study Group," *Lancet* 351, no. 9118 (1998): 1755–62.

12. ACCORD Study Group et al., "Effects of Intensive Blood-Pressure Control in Type 2 Diabetes Mellitus," *New England Journal of Medicine* 362 (2010): 1575–85.

13. SPRINT Research Group et al., "A Randomized Trial of Intensive versus Standard Blood-Pressure Control," *New England Journal of Medicine* 373 (2015): 2103–16.

14. P. A. James et al., "2014 Evidence-Based Guideline for the Management of High Blood Pressure in Adults: Report from the Panel Members Appointed to the Eight Joint National Committee (JNC 8)," *Journal of the American Medical Association* 311, no. 5 (2014): 507–20.

4. CHOLESTEROL

1. A. Keys, "Coronary Heart Disease in Seven Countries," *Circulation* 41, no. 4 (1970): I1–I211.

2. J. L. Goldstein and M. S. Brown, "Binding and Degradation of Low Density Lipoproteins by Cultured Human Fibroblasts: Comparison of Cells from a Normal Heart and from a Patient with Homozygous Familial Hypercholesterolemia," *Journal of Biological Chemistry* 249 (1974): 5153–62.

3. D. J. Rader, J. Cohen, and H. H. Hobbs, "Monogenic Hypercholesterolemia: New Insights in Pathogenesis and Treatment," *Journal of Clinical Investigation* 111, no. 12 (2003): 1795–803.

4. P. M. Ridker et al., "Rosuvastatin to Prevent Vascular Events in Men and Women with Elevated C-reactive Protein," *New England Journal of Medicine* 359 (2008): 2195–207.

5. C. P. Cannon et al., "Ezetimibe Added to Statin Therapy after Acute Coronary Syndromes," *New England Journal of Medicine* 372 (2015): 2387–97.

5. BLOOD CLOTS

1. S. P. Dehmer, M. V. Maciosek, T. J. Flottemesch, A. B. LaFrance, and E. P. Whitlock, "Aspirin for the Primary Prevention of Cardiovascular Disease and Colorectal Cancer: A Decision Analysis for the U.S. Preventive Services Task Force," *Annals of Internal Medicine* 164, no. 12 (2016): 777–86.

2. S. D. Wiviott et al., "Prasugrel versus Clopidogrel in Patients with Acute Coronary Syndromes," *New England Journal of Medicine* 357 (2007): 2001–15.

6. OBESITY

1. P. Nordstrom, N. L. Pedersen, Y. Gustafson, K. Michaelsson, and A. Nordstrom, "Risks of Myocardial Infarction, Death and Diabetes in Identical Twin Pairs with Different Body Mass Indexes," *JAMA Internal Medicine* 176, no. 10 (2016): 1522–29.

2. R. Furchgott, "The Discovery of Endothelium-Derived Relaxing Factor and Its Importance in the Identification of Nitric Oxide," *Journal of the American Medical Association* 276, no. 14 (1996): 1186–88; T. Munzel, C. Sinning, F. Post, A. Warnholtz, and E. Schulz, "Pathophysiology, Diagnosis and Prognostic Implications of Endothelial Dysfunction," *Annals of Medicine* 40, no. 3 (2008): 180–96; M. Gilani et al., "Role of Nitric Oxide Deficiency and Its Detection as a Risk Factor in Pre-hypertension," *Journal of the American Society of Hypertension* 1, no. 1 (2007): 45–55.

3. G. E. McVeigh, L. LeMay, D. Morgan, and J. N. Cohn, "Effects of Long-Term Cigarette Smoking on Endothelium-Dependent Responses in Humans," *American Journal of Cardiology* 78, no. 6 (1996): 668–72.

4. R. Vogel, M. Corretti, and G. Plotnick, "Effect of a Single High-Fat Meal on Endothelial Function in Healthy Subjects," *American Journal of Cardiology* 79, no. 3 (1997): 350–54.

5. A. Allam et al., "Atherosclerosis in Ancient Egyptian Mummies: The Horus Study," *JACC Cardiovascular Imaging* 4, no. 4 (2011): 315–27.

6. W. A. Murphy Jr., D. Z. Nedden, P. Gostner, R. Knapp, W. Recheis, and H. Seidler, "The Iceman: Discovery and Imaging," *Radiology* 226, no. 3 (2003): 614–29.

7. The Look AHEAD Reasearch Group, "Cardiovascular Effects of Intesive Lifestyle Intervention in Type 2 Diabetes," *New England Journal of Medicine* 369 (2013): 145–54.

7. DIABETES

1. C. L. Meinert, G. L. Knatterud, T. E. Prout, and C. R. Klimt, "A Study of the Effects of Hypoglycemic Agents on Vascular Complications in Patients with Adult-Onset Diabetes. II. Mortality Results," *Diabetes* 19 (1970): 747-830; The Diabetes Cont. and Comp. Trial Research Group, "The Effect of Intensive Treatment of Diabetes on the Development and Progression of Long-Term Complications in Insulin-Dependent Diabetes Mellitus," *New England Journal of Medicine* 329 (1993): 977–86; Prospective Diabetes Study Group, "Tight Blood Pres-

sure Control and Risk of Macrovascular and Microvascular Complications in Type 2 Diabetes: UKPDS 38," *British Medical Journal* 317 (1998): 703–17.

2. The Expert Committee on the Diagnosis and Classification of Diabetes Mellitus, "Follow-up Report on the Diagnosis of Diabetes Mellitus," *Diabetes Care* 26, no. 11 (2003): 3160–67.

3. D. J. Freeman et al., "Pravastatin and the Development of Diabetes Mellitus: Evidence for a Protective Treatment Effect in the West of Scotland Coronary Prevention Study," *Circulation* 103, no. 3 (2001): 357–62.

4. T. K. Schramm et al., "Diabetes Patients Requiring Glucose-Lowering Therapy and Nondiabetics with a Prior Myocardial Infarction Carry the Same Cardiovascular Risk: A Population Study of 3.3 Million People," *Circulation* 117, no. 15 (2008): 1945–54.

8. SMOKING

1. W. L. Watson and A. J. Conte, "Smoking and Lung Cancer," *Cancer* 7, no. 2 (1954): 245–49.

2. D. S. Celermajer et al., "Passive Smoking and Impaired Endothelium-Dependent Arterial Dilatation in Healthy Young Adults," *New England Journal of Medicine* 334 (1996): 150–54.

3. P. O. Bonetti, A. Lerman, and L. O. Lerman, "Endothelial Dysfunction: A Marker of Atherosclerotic Risk," *Arteriosclerosis, Thrombosis, and Vascular Biology* 23, no. 2 (2003): 168–75.

4. D. Harrison, K. Griendling, U. Landmesser, B. Hornig, and H. Drexler, "Role of Oxidative Stress in Atherosclerosis," *American Journal of Cardiology* 91, no. 3A (2003): 7–11.

9. DIET

1. A. O'Connor, "New Dietary Guidelines Urge Less Sugar for All and Less Protein for Boys and Men," *New York Times*, January 7, 2016.

2. J. Cawley and C. Meyerhoefer, "The Medical Care Costs of Obesity: An Instrumental Variables Approach," *Journal of Health Econonmics* 31, no. 1 (2012): 219–30.

3. S. Kenchaiah et al., "Obesity and the Risk of Heart Failure," *New England Journal of Medicine* 347 (2002): 305–13.

4. C. J. Lavie, M. A. Alpert, R. Arena, M. R. Mehra, R. V. Milani, and H. O. Ventura, "Impact of Obesity and the Obesity Paradox on Prevalence and Prognosis in Heart Failure," *JACC Heart Failure* 1, no. 2 (2013): 93–102.

5. M. H. Weinberger, "Salt Sensitivity of Blood Pressure in Humans," *Hypertension* 27, no. 3 (1996): 481–90.

6. R. D. Sembra et al., "Resveratrol Levels and All-Cause Mortality in Older Community-Dwelling Adults," *JAMA Internal Medicine* 174, no. 7 (2014): 1077–84.

7. T. S. Rector et al., "Ramndomized, Double-Blind, Placebo-Controlled Study of Supplemental Oral L-arginine in Patients with Heart Failure," *Circulation* 93, no. 12 (1996): 2135–41.

10. INFLAMMATION

1. P. Libby, P. M. Ridker, and A. Maseri, "Inflammation and Atherosclerosis," *Circulation* 105 (2002): 1135–43; G. K. Hansson, "Inflammation, Atherosclerosis, and Coronary Artery Disease," *New England Journal of Medicine* 352, no. 16 (2005): 1685–95.

2. P. M. Ridker, J. W. Buring, N. Rifai, and N. R. Cook, "Development and Validation of Improved Algorithms for the Assessment of Global Cardiovascular Risk in Women: The Reynolds Risk Score," *Journal of the American Medical Association* 297, no. 6 (2007): 611–19.

3. M. Gopal, A. Bhaskaran, W. I. Khalife, and A. Barbagelata, "Heart Disease in Patients with HIV/AIDS—An Emerging Clinical Problem," *Current Cardiology Reviews* 5, no. 2 (2009): 149–54.

4. S. Van Doornum, G. McColl, and I. P. Wicks, "Accelerated Atherosclerosis: An Extraarticular Feature of Rheumatoid Arthritis?" *Arthritis & Rheumatology* 46, no. 4 (2002): 862–73.

5. M. Bäck and G. K. Hansson, "Anti-inflammatory Therapies for Atherosclerosis," *Nature Reviews Cardiology* 12 (2015): 199–211.

11. STATISTICS VERSUS BIOLOGY

1. "ICD-ICD10-CM-International Classification of Diseases," *Clinical Modification*, n.d.

2. S. H. Woolf, R. Grol, A. Hutchinson, M. Eccles, and J. Grimshaw, "Potential Benefits, Limitations, and Harms of Clinical Guidelines," *British Medical Journal* 318 (1999): 527–30.

3. J. N. Cohn, "The Fallacy of the Mean," *Journal of Cardiac Failure* 7, no. 2 (2001): 103–4.

12. DETECTION OF EARLY DISEASE

1. D. Mozaffarian et al., "American Heart Association Statistics Committee and Stroke Statistics Subcommittee: Heart Disease and Stroke Statistics—2015 Update: A Report from the American Heart Association," *Circulation* 131 (2015): e29–322.

2. D. M. Lloyd-Jones, Y. Hong, D. Labarthe, D. Mozaffarian, L. J. Appel, L. van Horn, K. Greenlund, S. Daniels, C. Nichol, G. F. Tomaselli, D. K. Arnett, G. C. Fonarow, P. M. Ho, M. S. Lauer, F. A. Masoudi, R. M. Robertson, V. Roger, L. H. Schwamm, P. Sorlie, C. W. Yancy, W. D. Rosamond, and American Heart Association Strategic Planning Task Force and Statistics Committee, "Defining and Setting National Goals for Cardiovascular Health Promotion and Disease Reduction: The American Heart Association's Strategic Impact Goal through 2020 and Beyond," *Circulation* 121 (2010): 586–613.

3. A. V. Khera, C. A. Emdin, I. Drake, P. Natarajan, A. G. Bick, N. R. Cook, D. I. Chasman, U. Baber, R. Mehran, D. J. Rader, V. Fuster, E. Boerwinkle, O. Melander, M. Orho-Melander, P. M. Ridker, and S. Kathiresan, "Genetic Risk, Adherence to a Healthy Lifestyle, and Coronary Disease," *New England Journal of Medicine* 375 (2016): 2349–58.

4. A. Keller et al., "New Insights into the Tyrolean Iceman's Origin and Phenotype as Inferred by Whole-Genome Sequencing," *Nature Communications* 3 (2012): 698.

5. M. D. Miedema, J. N. Cohn, R. F. Garberich, T. Knickelbine, K. J. Graham, and T. D. Henry, "Underuse of Cardiovascular Preventive Pharmacotherapy in Patients Presenting with ST-Elevation Myocardial Infarction," *American Heart Journal* 164, no. 2 (2012): 259–67.

6. D. A. Duprez et al., "Vascular and Cardiac Functional and Structural Screening to Identify Risk of Future Morbid Events: Preliminary Observations," *Journal of the American Society of Hypertension* 5, no. 5 (2011): 401–9.

7. D. A. Duprez, N. D. Florea, K. Jones, and J. N. Cohn, "Beneficial Effects of Valsartan in Asymptomatic Individuals with Vascular or Cardiac Abnormalities: The DETECTIV Pilot Study," *Journal of the American College of Cardiology* 50, no. 9 (2007): 835–39; S. M. Saul, D. A. Duprez, W. Zhong, G. A. Grandits, and J. N. Cohn, "Effect of Carvedilol, Lisinopril, and Their Combination on Vascular and Cardiac Health in Patients with Borderline Blood Pressure: The DETECT Study," *Journal of Human Hypertension* 27, no. 6 (2013): 362–67.

13. SECONDARY PREVENTION

1. R. B. D'Agostino Sr., R. S. Vasan, M. J. Pencina, P. A. Wolf, M. Cobain, and J. M. Massaro,"General Cardiovascular Risk Profile for Use in Primary Care: The Framingham Heart Study," *Circulation* 117, no. 6 (2008): 743–53.

2. Heart Association Task Force on Practice Guidelines, "2013 ACC/AHA Guideline on the Assessment of Cardiovascular Risk: A Report of the American College of Cardiology/American Heart Association Task Force on Practice Guidelines," *Circulation* 129 (2014): S49–73.

3. J. S. Forrester et al., "27th Bethesda Conference: Matching the Intensity of Risk Factor Management with the Hazard for Coronary Disease Events. Task Force 4. Efficacy of Risk Factor Management," *Journal of the American College of Cardiology* 27, no. 5 (1996): 991–1006.

4. J. N. Cohn et al., "Screening for Early Detection of Cardiovascular Disease in Asymptomatic Individuals," *American Heart Journal* 146, no. 4 (2003): 679–85.

14. A COMMUNITY APPROACH

1. J. N. Cohn et al., "Noninvasive Pulse Wave Analysis for the Detection of Arterial Vascular Disease," *Hypertension* 26, no. 3 (1995): 503–8.

2. J. N. Cohn et al., "Coadministered Amlodopine and Atorvastatin Produces Early Improvements in Arterial Wall Compliance in Hypertensive Patients with Dyslipidemia," *American Journal of Hypertension* 22, no. 2 (2009): 137–44.

15. A FUTURE FREE OF SYMPTOMATIC CARDIOVASCULAR DISEASE

1. B. Dahlöf et al., "Prevention of Cardiovascular Events with an Antihypertensive Regimen of Amlodipine Adding Perindopril as Required versus Atenolol Adding Bendroflumethiazide as Required, in the Anglo-Scandinavian Cardiac Outcomes Trial-Blood Pressure Lowering Arm (ASCOT-BPLA): A Multicentre Randomised Controlled Trial," *Lancet* 366, no. 9489 (2005): 895–906.

2. Cholesterol Treatment Trialists' (CTT) Collaboration et al., "Efficacy and Safety of More Intensive Lowering LDL Cholesterol: A Meta-analysis of Data from 170,000 Participants in 26 Randomised Trials," *Lancet* 376, no. 9753 (2010): 1670–81.

BIBLIOGRAPHY

ACCORD Study Group et al. "Effects of Intensive Blood-Pressure Control in Type 2 Diabetes Mellitus." *New England Journal of Medicine* 362 (2010): 1575–85.

Allam, A., et al. "Atherosclerosis in Ancient Egyptian Mummies: The Horus Study." *JACC Cardiovascular Imaging* 4, no. 4 (2011): 315–27.

Alpert, J. S., K. Thygesen, E. Antman, and J. P. Bassand. "Myocardial Infarction Redefined— A Consensus Document of the Joint European Society of Cardiology/American College of Cardiology Committee for the Redefinition of Myocardial Infarction." *Journal of the American College of Cardiology* 36, no. 3 (2000): 959–69.

Altman, L. K. "Drug Used in Emergencies Depsite Warnings." *New York Times*, October 23, 1996.

Antman, E. M., et al. "ACC/AHA Guidelines for the Management of Patients with ST-Elevation Myocardial Infarction; A Report of the American College of Cardiology/American Heart Association Task Force on Practice Guidelines (Committee to Revise the 1999 Guidelines for the Management of Patients with Acute Myocardial Infarction." *Journal of the American College of Cardiology* 44, no. 3 (2004): E1–E211.

Bäck, M., and Hansson, G. K. "Anti-inflammatory Therapies for Atherosclerosis." *Nature Reviews Cardiology* 12 (2015): 199–211.

Bairey Merz, C. N. "Women and Ischemic Heart Disease Paradox and Pathophysiology." *JACC Cardiovascular Imaging* 4, no. 1 (2011): 74–77.

Bonetti, P. O., Lerman, A., and Lerman, L. O. "Endothelial Dysfunction: A Marker of Atherosclerotic Risk." *Arteriosclerosis, Thrombosis, and Vascular Biology* 23, no. 2 (2003): 168–75.

Booth, J. "A Short History of Blood Pressure Measurement." *Proceedings of the Royal Society of Medicine* 70, no. 11 (1977): 793–99.

Cannon, C. P., et al. "Ezetimibe Added to Statin Therapy after Acute Coronary Syndromes." *New England Journal of Medicine* 372 (2015): 2387–97.

Cawley, J., and Meyerhoefer, C. "The Medical Care Costs of Obesity: An Instrumental Variables Approach." *Journal of Health Economics* 31, no.1 (2012): 219–30.

Celermajer, D. S., et al. "Passive Smoking and Impaired Endothelium-Dependent Arterial Dilatation in Healthy Young Adults." *New England Journal of Medicine* 334 (1996): 150–54.

Chobanian, A. V., et al. "The Seventh Report of the Joint National Committee on Prevention, Detection, Evaluation and Treatment of High Blood Pressure: The JNC 7 report." *Journal of the American Medical Association* 289, no. 19 (2003): 2560–72.

Cholesterol Treatment Trialists' Collaboration, et al. "Efficacy and Safety of More Intensive Lowering LDL Cholesterol: A Meta-analysis of Data from 170,000 Participants in 26 Randomised Trials." *Lancet* 376, no. 9753 (2010): 1670–81.

Cohn, J. N. "The fallacy of the mean." *Journal of Cardiac Failure* 7, no. 2 (2001): 103–4.

Cohn, J. N., et al. "Coadministered Amlodopine and Atorvastatin Produces Early Improvements in Arterial Wall Compliance in Hypertensive Patients with Dyslipidemia." *American Journal of Hypertension* 22, no. 2 (2009): 137–44.

Cohn, J. N., et al. "Noninvasive Pulse Wave Analysis for the Detection of Arterial Vascular Disease." *Hypertension* 26, no. 3 (1995): 503–8.

Cohn, J. N., et al. "Screening for Early Detection of Cardiovascular Disease in Asymptomatic Individuals." *American Heart Journal* 146, no. 4 (2003): 679–85.

D'Agostino Sr., R. B., R. S. Vasan, M. J. Pencina, P. A. Wolf, M. Cobain, and J. M. Massaro. "General Cardiovascular Risk Profile for Use in Primary Care: The Framingham Heart Study." *Circulation* 117, no. 6 (2008): 743–53.

Dahlöf, B., et al. "Prevention of Cardiovascular Events with an Antihypertensive Regimen of Amlodipine Adding Perindopril as Required versus Atenolol Adding Bendroflumethiazide as Required, in the ASCOT-BPLA Trial: A Multicentre Randomised Controlled Trial." *Lancet* 366, no. 9489 (2005): 895–906.

Dehmer, S. P., M. V. Maciosek, T. J. Flottemesch, A. B. LaFrance, and E. P. Whitlock. "Aspirin for the Primary Prevention of Cardiovascular Disease and Colorectal Cancer: A Decision Analysis for the U.S. Preventive Services Task Force." *Annals of Internal Medicine* 164, no. 12 (2016): 777–86.

Diabetes Cont. and Comp. Trial Research Group. "The Effect of Intensive Treatment of Diabetes on the Development and Progression of Long-Term Complications in Insulin-Dependent Diabetes Mellitus." *New England Journal of Medicine* 329 (1993): 977–86.

Diagnostic and Statistical Manual of Mental Disorders (DSM-5). Washington, DC: American Psychiatric Association, 2013.

Dorland, W. A. Newman. *Dorland's Medical Dictionary.* Philadelphia: Elsevier/Saunders, 2011.

Duprez, D. A., et al. "Determinants of Radial Artery Pulse Wave Analysis in Asymptomatic Individuals." *American Journal of Hypertension* 17, no. 8 (2004): 647–53.

Duprez, D. A., et al. "Vascular and Cardiac Functional and Structural Screening to Identify Risk of Future Morbid Events: Preliminary Observations." *Journal of the American Society of Hypertension* 5, no. 5 (2011): 401–9.

Duprez, D. A., N. D. Florea, K. Jones, and J. N. Cohn. "Beneficial Effects of Valsartan in Asymptomatic Individuals with Vascular or Cardiac Abnormalities: The DETECTIV Pilot Study." *Journal of the American College of Cardiology* 50, no. 9 (2007): 835–39.

Enos, W. F., R. H. Homes, and J. Beyer. "Coronary Disease among United States Soldiers Killed in Action in Korea; Preliminary Report." *Journal of the American Medical Association* 152, no. 12 (1953): 1090–93.

Ettehad, D., et al. "Blood Pressure Lowering for Prevention of Cardiovascular Disease and Death: A Systematic Review and Meta-analysis." *Lancet* 387, no. 10022 (2016): 957–67.

Expert Committee on the Diagnosis and Classification of Diabetes Mellitus. "Follow-up Report on the Diagnosis of Diabetes Mellitus." *Diabetes Care* 26, no. 11 (2003): 3160–67.

Forrester, J. S., et al. "27th Bethesda Conference: Matching the Intensity of Risk Factor Management with the Hazard for Coronary Disease Events. Task Force 4. Efficacy of Risk Factor Management." *Journal of the American College of Cardiology* 27, no. 5 (1996): 991–1006.

Frank, Sanders T. "Aural Sign of Coronary Artery Disease." *New England Journal of Medicine* 289, no. 6 (1973): 327–28.

Franklin, S. S. "Ageing and Hypertension: The Assessment of Blood Pressure Indices in Predicting Coronary Heart Disease." *Journal of Hypertension Supplement* 17, no. 5 (1999): S29–36.

Freeman, D. J., et al. "Pravastatin and the Development of Diabetes Mellitus: Evidence for a Protective Treatment Effect in the West of Scotland Coronary Prevention Study." *Circulation* 103, no. 3 (2001): 357–62.

Friedberg, C. K. *Diseases of the Heart.* 2nd ed. Philadelphia: W. B. Saunders Company, 1956.

Furchgott, R. "The Discovery of Endothelium-Derived Relaxing Factor and Its Importance in the Identification of Nitric Oxide." *Journal of the American Medical Association* 276, no. 14 (1996): 1186–88.

Gerdes, A. M., et al. "Structural Remodeling of Cardiac Myocytes in Patients with Ischemic Cardiomyopathy." *Circulation* 86, no. 2 (1992): 426–30.

Gilani, M., et al. "Role of Nitric Oxide Deficiency and Its Detection as a Risk Factor in Pre-hypertension." *Journal of the American Society of Hypertension* 1, no. 1 (2007): 45–55.

GISSI (Gruppo Italiano per lo Studio Della Streptochinasi Nell'Infarto Miocardico). "Effectiveness of Intravenous Thrombolytic Treatment in Acute Myocardial Infarction." *Lancet* 1, no. 8478 (1986): 397–402.

Go, A. S., et al. "Heart Disease and Stroke Statistics—2013 Update: A Report from the American Heart Association." *Circulation* 127, no. 1 (2013): e6–e245.

Goldstein, J. L., and Brown, M. S. "Binding and Degradation of Low Density Lipoproteins by Cultured Human Fibroblasts: Comparison of Cells from a Normal Heart and from a Patient with Homozygous Familial Hypercholesterolemia." *Journal of Biological Chemistry* 249 (1974): 5153–62.

Gopal, M., A. Bhaskaran, W. I. Khalife, and A. Barbagelata. "Heart Disease in Patients with HIV/AIDS—An Emerging Clinical Problem." *Current Cardiology Reviews* 5, no. 2 (2009): 149–54.

Hall, W. D. "Stephen Hales: Theologian, Botanist, Physiologist, Discoverer of Hemodynamics." *Clinical Cardiology* 10, no. 8 (1987): 487–89.

Hansson, G. K. "Inflammation, Atherosclerosis, and Coronary Artery Disease." *New England Journal of Medicine* 352, no. 16 (2005): 1685–95.

Hansson, L., et al. "Effects of Intensive Blood-Pressure Lowering and Low-Dose Aspirin in Patients with Hypertension: Principal Results of the Hypertension Optimal Treatment (HOT) Randomised Trial, HOT Study Group." *Lancet* 351, no. 9118 (1998): 1755–62.

Harrison, D., K. Griendling, U. Landmesser, B. Hornig, and H. Drexler. "Role of Oxidative Stress in Atherosclerosis." *American Journal of Cardiology* 91, no. 3A (2003): 7–11.

Heart Association Task Force on Practice Guidelines. "2013 ACC/AHA Guideline on the Assessment of Cardiovascular Risk: A Report of the American College of Cardiology/ American Heart Association Task Force on Practice Guidelines." *Circulation* 129 (2014): S49–73.

"ICD-ICD10-CM-International Classification of Diseases." *Clinical Modification.* n.d.

James, P. A., et al. "2014 Evidence-Based Guideline for the Management of High Blood Pressure in Adults: Report from the Panel Members Appointed to the Eighth Joint National Committee (JNC 8)." *Journal of the American Medical Association* 311, no. 5 (2014): 507–20.

Keller, A., et al. "New Insights into the Tyrolean Iceman's Origin and Phenotype as Inferred by Whole-Genome Sequencing." *Nature Communications* 3 (2012): 698.

Kenchaiah, S., et al. "Obesity and the risk of heart failure." *New England Journal of Medicine,* 347 (2002): 305–13.

Keys, A. "Coronary Heart Disease in Seven Countries." *Circulation* 41, no. 4 (1970): I1–I211.

Khera, A. V., et al. "Genetic Risk, Adherence to a Healthy Lifestyle, and Coronary Disease." *New England Journal of Medicine* 375 (2016): 2349–58.

Krumholz, H. M., et al. "Reduction in Acute Myocardial Infarction Mortality in the United States: Risk-Standardized Mortality Rates from 1995–2006." *Journal of the American Medical Association* 302, no. 7 (2009): 767–73.

Lavie, C. J., M. A. Alpert, R. Arena, M. R. Mehra, R. V. Milani, and H. O. Ventura. "Impact of Obesity and the Obesity Paradox on Prevalence and Prognosis in Heart Failure." *JACC Heart Failure* 1, no. 2 (2013): 93–102.

Lewington, S., R. Clarke, N. Qizilbash, R. Peto, R. Collins, and Prospective Studies Collaboration. "Age-Specific Relevance of Usual Blood Pressure to Vascular Mortality: A Meta-analysis of Individual Data for One Million Adults in 61 Prospective Studies." *Lancet* 360, no. 9349 (2002): 1903–13.

Libby, P., P. M. Ridker, and A. Maseri. "Inflammation and Atherosclerosis." *Circulation* 105 (2002): 1135–43.

Linzbach, A. J. "Heart Failure from the Point of View of Quantitative Anatomy." *American Journal of Cardiology* 5 (1960): 370–82.

Lloyd-Jones, D. M., et al. "Defining and Setting National Goals for Cardiovascular Health Promotion and Disease Reduction: The American Heart Association's Strategic Impact Goal through 2020 and Beyond." *Circulation* 121 (2010): 586–613.

Lloyd-Jones, D. M., et al. "Prediction of Lifetime Risk for Cardiovascular Disease by Risk Factor Burden at 50 Years of Age." *Circulation* 113 (2006): 791–98.

Look AHEAD Reasearch Group. "Cardiovascular Effects of Intesive Lifestyle Intervention in Type 2 Diabetes." *New England Journal of Medicine* 369 (2013): 145–54.

McVeigh, G. E., L. LeMay, D. Morgan, and J. N. Cohn. "Effects of Long-Term Cigarette Smoking on Endothelium-Dependent Responses in Humans." *American Journal of Cardiology* 78, no. 6 (1996): 668–72.

Meinert, C. L., G. L. Knatterud, T. E. Prout, and C. R. Klimt. "A Study of the Effects of Hypoglycemic Agents on Vascular Complications in Patients with Adult-Onset Diabetes. II. Mortality Results." *Diabetes* 19 (1970): 747–830.

Miedema, M. D., J. N. Cohn, R. F. Garberich, T. Knickelbine, K. J. Graham, and T. D. Henry. "Underuse of Cardiovascular Preventive Pharmacotherapy in Patients Presenting with ST-Elevation Myocardial Infarction." *American Heart Journal* 164, no. 2 (2012): 259–67.

Mozaffarian, D., et al. "American Heart Association Statistics Commitee and Stroke Statistics Subcommittee: Heart Disease and Stroke Statistics—2015 Update: A Report from the American Heart Association." *Circulation* 131 (2015): e29–322.

Munzel, T., C. Sinning, F. Post, A. Warnholtz, and E. Schulz. "Pathophysiology, Diagnosis and Prognostic Implications of Endothelial Dysfunction." *Annals of Medicine* 40, no. 3 (2008): 180–96.

Murphy, W. A., Jr., D. Z. Nedden, P. Gostner, R. Knapp, W. Recheis, and H. Seidler. "The Iceman: Discovery and Imaging." *Radiology* 226, no. 3 (2003): 614–29.

Naghavi, M., et al. "From Vulnerable Plaque to Vulnerable Patient: A Call for New Definitions and Risk Assessment Strategies: Part I." *Circulation* 108, no. 14 (2003): 1664–72.

Nordstrom, P., N. L. Pedersen, Y. Gustafson, K. Michaelsson, and A. Nordstrom. "Risks of Myocardial Infarction, Death and Diabetes in Identical Twin Pairs with Different Body Mass Indexes." *JAMA Internal Medicine* 176, no. 10 (2016): 1522–29.

O'Connor, A. "New Dietary Guidelines Urge Less Sugar for All and Less Protein for Boys and Men." *New York Times*, January 7, 2016.

O'Rourke, M. F. *Arterial Function in Health and Disease.* London: Churchill Livingston, 1982.

"Prevention of Stroke by Antihypertensive Drug Treatment in Older Persons with Isolated Systolic Hypertension: Final Results of the Systolic Hypertension in Elderly Program (SHEP), SHEP Cooperative Research Group." *Journal of the American Medical Association* 265, no. 24 (1991): 3255–64.

Prospective Diabetes Study Group. "Tight Blood Pressure Control and Risk of Macrovascular and Microvascular Complications in Type 2 Diabetes: UKPDS 38." *British Medical Journal* 317 (1998): 703–17.

Rader, D. J., J. Cohen, and H. H. Hobbs. "Monogenic Hypercholesterolemia: New Insights in Pathogenesis and Treatment." *Journal of Clinical Investigation* 111, no. 12 (2003): 1795–803.

Rector, T. S., et al. "Ramndomized, Double-Blind, Placebo-Controlled Study of Supplemental Oral L-arginine in Patients with Heart Failure." *Circulation* 93, no. 12 (1996): 2135–41.

Ridker, P. M., J. W. Buring, N. Rifai, and M. R. Cook. "Development and Validation of Improved Algorithms for the Assessment of Global Cardiovascular Risk in Women: The Reynolds Risk Score." *Journal of the American Medical Association* 297, no. 6 (2007): 611–19.

Ridker, P. M., et al. "Rosuvastatin to Prevent Vascular Events in Men and Women with Elevated C-reactive Protein." *New England Journal of Medicine* 359 (2008): 2195–207.

Safar, Michel E., and Gerard M. London. "Arterial and Venous Compliance in Sustained Essential Hypertension." *Hypertension* 10, no. 2 (1987): 133–39.

Saul, S. M., D. A. Duprez, W. Zhong, G. A. Grandits, and J. N. Cohn. "Effect of Carvedilol, Lisinopril, and Thier Combination on Vascular and Cardiac Health in Patients with Borderline Blood Pressure: The DETECT Study." *Journal of Human Hypertension* 27, no. 6 (2013): 362–67.

Schramm, T. K., et al. "Diabetes Patients Requiring Glucose-Lowering Therapy and Nondiabetics with a Prior Myocardial Infarction Carry the Same Cardiovascular Risk: A Population Study of 3.3 Million People." *Circulation* 117, no. 15 (2008): 1945–54.

Sembra, R. D., et al. "Resveratrol Levels and All-Cause Mortality in Older Community-Dwelling Adults." *JAMA Internal Medicine* 174, no. 7 (2014): 1077–84.

SPRINT Research Group et al. "A Randomized Trial of Intensive versus Standard Blood-Pressure Control." *New England Journal of Medicine* 373 (2015): 2103–16.

Swedberg, K., et al. "Treatment of Anemia with Darbepoetin Alfa in Systolic Heart Failure." *New England Journal of Medicine* 368 (2013): 1210–19.

Templin, C., et al. "Clinical Features and Outcomes of Takotsubo (Stress) Cardiomyopathy." *New England Journal of Medicine* 373 (2015): 929–38.

VA Coop Study. "Effects of Treatment on Morbidity in Hypertension. II. Results in Patients with Diastolic Blood Pressure Averaging 90 through 114 mm Hg." *Journal of the American Medical Association* 213, no. 7 (1970): 1143–52.

Van Doornum, S., G. McColl, and I. P. Wicks. "Accelerated Atherosclerosis: An Extraarticular Feature of Rheumatoid Arthritis?" *Arthritis & Rheumatology* 46, no. 4 (2002): 862–73.

Vasan, R. S., et al. "Impact of High-Normal Blood Pressure on the Risk of Cardiovascular Disease." *New England Journal of Medicine* 345, no. 18 (2001): 1291–97.

Vogel, R., M. Corretti, and G. Plotnick. "Effect of a Single High-Fat Meal on Endothelial Function in Healthy Subjects." *American Journal of Cardiology* 79, no. 3 (1997): 350–54.

Watson, W. L., and Conte, A. J. "Smoking and Lung Cancer." *Cancer* 7, no. 2 (1954): 245–49.

Weinberger, M. H. "Salt Sensitivity of Blood Pressure in Humans." *Hypertension* 27, no. 3 (1996): 481–90.

Wiviott, S. D., et al. "Prasugrel versus Clopidogrel in Patients with Acute Coronary Syndromes." *New England Journal of Medicine* 357 (2007): 2001–15.

Woolf, S. H., R. Grol, A. Hutchinson, M. Eccles, and J. Grimshaw. "Potential Benefits, Limitations, and Harms of Clinical Guidelines." *British Medical Journal* 318 (1999): 527–30.

INDEX

ABOUT THE AUTHOR

Jay N. Cohn, MD, is professor of medicine at the University of Minnesota Medical School and director of the Rasmussen Center for Cardiovascular Disease Prevention. He was director of the university's Cardiovascular Division from 1974 to 1996. He is widely recognized for his contributions to the understanding and management of hypertension, coronary artery disease, myocardial infarction, and heart failure. He is the author of the scientific memoir *Saving Sam: Drugs, Race, and Discovering the Secrets of Heart Disease.* He has published over 750 scientific papers and has been honored for his research accomplishments by the American Heart Association, American College of Cardiology, American College of Physicians, American Society of Hypertension, Heart Failure Society of America, American Association for the Advancement of Science, Cornell University, and the University of Minnesota. He has served as president of four national and international societies and is co-editor of a major textbook, *Cardiovascular Medicine.* He holds a number of patents on devices and drugs used to diagnose and treat cardiovascular disease.